Anaesthesia for Vascular Surgery

Anaesthesia for Vascular Surgery

P. J. Tomlin MB BS, FFARCS

Late Consultant Anaesthetist
Queen Elizabeth Hospital, Birmingham
Senior Clinical Lecturer
University of Birmingham

WRIGHT

London   Boston   Durban   Singapore   Sydney   Toronto   Wellington

John Wright
is an imprint of Butterworth Scientific

First published 1988

© **Butterworth & Co. (Publishers) Ltd, 1988**

British Library Cataloguing in Publication Data

Tomlin, P. J.
    Anaesthesia for vascular surgery.
    1. Anesthesia   2. Blood-vessels
    I. Title
    617′.967413   RD87.3.B/

ISBN 0 7236 0831 8

Photoset by Bath Typesetting Ltd
Printed and bound by Billing and Sons Ltd, Worcester

Dedication

This book is dedicated to all my colleagues in the University Department of Surgery, Birmingham, England with affection and in appreciation of many exciting and happy years of collaboration with them as a vascular anaesthetist.

Preface

With the increasing number of people achieving advanced years, vascular surgery has become one of the major growth areas of modern surgery. Twenty years ago abdominal aneurysmectomy was a rare event; now it is commonplace. Yet anaesthesia for vascular surgery is among the most demanding branches of the specialty. To do it well is among the most exacting and professionally satisfying of all tasks that face the modern anaesthetist. It has its drama, indeed great drama, and alas, its disappointments for this is high-risk anaesthesia and high-risk surgery, but to do it well requires both the art and the science of anaesthesia. In this particular field, as in no other, the art must be based on the science. Science can be taught or acquired from books, but the art must be learnt and learnt from experience, tempered with knowledge, at the operating table.

Vascular anaesthetists must liaise closely with the surgical team, for above all else vascular surgery is teamwork and an effective team requires understanding of each other's problems. It is only out of this collaboration that improved results come. Unlike many other branches of surgery, vascular surgeons have tended to be ahead of their time in striving for the clinically impossible. A simple example is Langenbeck, nearly a century ago, attempting pulmonary embolectomy before the days of endotracheal intubation, let alone controlled ventilation. Yet, to the vascular surgeon the situation is starkly simple. Unless the operation is performed, novel though it might be, the patient will die or perhaps be condemned to a twilight world *sans* legs in advancing years and desperately dependent upon the good-will of others for the simple amenities of living. In such a situation, to save a limb is to save a life. In rising to meet this need, the surgeon challenges the anaesthetist—can he keep this patient, who is not the fittest of patients, alive and free from pain and in such good condition to suffer what might be among the most massive of surgical assaults and, finally, return the patient back to him, preferably in a better condition than when he first presented? Then, just when the anaesthetist learns to achieve the apparently clinically impossible, the surgeon throws him yet another challenge: suprarenal aneurysms were virtually untreatable ten years ago. Not now though!

This book has been written to serve several purposes. Its prime purpose is to provide the knowledge, in particular of applied physiology, necessary for the understanding of anaesthesia for vascular surgery. A background knowledge of basic sciences and physiology up to the level of the Primary FFARCS examination is assumed, although key components are revised briefly where appropriate. This book should contain enough to meet all the demands of the Final FFARCS examination as far as anaesthesia for vascular surgery is concerned, and hopefully contains much more.

The book is not written as a recipe book, telling you when to do this or that. Nevertheless, its purpose is to serve as a bench book that can be consulted for discussion and ideas of the principles involved as to why such a particular event is likely to happen at such a particular stage. From knowledge of the principles involved the anaesthetist can then draw his own conclusions as to how to resolve a particular problem. To this end, the list of contents is unusually detailed. For the sake of clarity and brevity, scientific references have been kept to a minimum and a somewhat didactic style has been assumed, deliberately and as a challenge, in the hope of stimulating some thinking and perhaps rethinking of the principles involved in patient care during vascular surgery.

Two themes pervade this book throughout: an understanding of the principles of circulatory physiology as applied to the vascular surgery patient and the principles involved in the management of pain. It is the latter that offers the greatest challenge, where our scientific knowledge is weakest and our treatment mainly empirical, although the situation is rapidly improving. Unlike circulatory physiology, pain defies measurement and quantification, although many studies using analogue scales and indices have been and are being made. No apology is made for the constant reiteration of these two themes, for it is the compassionate response to pain that defines the humane anaesthetist and the appropriate use of applied circulatory physiology that defines the good anaesthetist in the field of vascular surgery or, for that matter, in any field of anaesthesia.

Although this book is primarily for the anaesthetist involved in vascular surgery, yet much of what applies to the vascular patient also applies to patients in other fields of surgery. In general surgery, in the United Kingdom, over fifty per cent of the patients are either retired or approaching retirement. Vascular disease is primarily a disease of degeneration and, inevitably, among the general surgical patients there will be many patients with varying disorders of the cardiovascular system. The principles of patient care, described in this book, also apply just as well to those patients as they do to the patient who is undergoing vascular surgery.

However, good patient care does not end when the nitrous oxide is discontinued. The last chapter concentrates on postoperative care. Here too the anaesthetist can and should play a significant role which can only be to the patient's benefit. Here too the emphasis must be on team work, team work between the anaesthetist and surgeon.

In the second paragraph of the last chapter appear the following words:

Vascular surgery is high-risk surgery. Twenty years ago the mortality after elective surgery for aneurysms was 10%, ten years ago it was about 5%. This improvement is largely due to better postoperative care. Nowadays an uncomplicated aneurysm carries with it a mortality of around 3%.... Emergency aortic surgery has a mortality rate that ranges from 37% to 69% with a mean of 54%. The bulk of this mortality occurs postoperatively. The mortality rate is very high in the initial postoperative period but then falls away. (See p. 194.)

There too lies another challenge.

P. J. T.

Contents

CHAPTER 1

Circulatory Considerations and Changes Consequent upon Arterial Disease

The conventional view of the circulation is that of the heart acting as a pump, pumping out a simple fluid into a large but rigid tube of negligible resistance until that fluid reaches the arterioles. Here it meets its main resistance and it is this resistance that determines the magnitude of the arterial pressure. The fluid is collected from the capillaries and flows back to the heart, being driven primarily by the residual pressure (*vis a tergo*) left after the fluid has overcome the resistance offered by the arterioles. Flow is thought of as being mainly laminar in type and occurring only during systole. This conception is too simplistic, to the point where it materially distorts the understanding required of the haemodynamics involved particularly in patients with arterial disease. Thus the systolic blood pressure is not governed by the degree of arteriolar tone generating a resistance, so that the pressure rises with the heart acted on by the feedback loop of the staircase response. (In this response the heart works harder when it meets a resistance; O'Rourke, 1982a.) Rather, in patients with severe arterial disease, the systolic blood pressure is governed much more by the extent of the aortic impedance (O'Rourke, 1982b). Even more importantly in such patients, hypotension is rarely due to changes in arteriolar tone, whether produced by anaesthetic agents or other drugs. It is much more commonly due to changes in myocardial contractility or to a failing venous return, or to both. This has important connotations in the clinical management of patients undergoing arterial surgery.

The circulation is an almost closed system consisting of the heart rhythmically pumping a non-Newtonian fluid through a series of conical elastic arteries with differing branching angles and variable degrees of elasticity. The tubes steadily proliferate in number but decrease in size, ending in a network that is a mixture of series and parallel circuits, only for these to rejoin to form progressively larger but fewer vessels ending with the vena cava. Blood flows through these tubes at variable rates of flow and pressure, dictated in part by the branching angle but principally by the diameter and number of the orifices to the capillary bed, that is the arterioles. The effects of branching and the branching angle are twofold. (1) If the branching angle incident to the flow is significantly greater than 130 degrees there is the danger that the branch will act as a Venturi device, particularly if the main line flow is at a high velocity. (2) If the run-off down the branch allows for a substantial flow, there will be turbulence at the origin of the branch. The effects of the turbulence in turn are twofold: it reduces mean flow and it imposes mechanical stresses on the intimal lining so that it eventually becomes a site for atheromatous deposition. This is well seen in the aorta in those zones of the aorta which contain large branches such as the subdiaphragmatic portion of the aorta or the aortic arch.

The system is not entirely closed. Some of the fluid that is circulated escapes only to be recaptured by the lymphatics and returned to the circulation via the thoracic duct. Some escapes through the glomerular tufts of the kidney only to be recaptured in part by the renal collecting tubules. There are a number of regional variations, some of which have substantial flows such as the portal system, others are minor such as the hypothesial portal system that drains the pituitary gland. Significant quantities of fluid are circulated by other means such as within the bowel, where secretion is high in the upper bowel but absorption predominates in the distal bowel.

Severe vascular disease produces changes which may significantly modify this overall pattern. The reduction in elasticity in the larger tubes materially affects the flow and pressure profiles within these vessels (Hardung, 1962). Irregular randomly scattered patches of atheroma also affect localized flow distribution and localized pressure gradients, whilst occlusive vascular disease may reduce substantially the size of the vascular bed, either locally or regionally, to the point of zero flow or dry gangrene.

THE FUNCTIONAL EFFICIENCY OF THE HEART

The heart consists of two pairs of muscular chambers attached either side of a tough fibrous skeleton. This skeleton is formed out of the rings which surround the heart valves and orifices of the great vessels. In normal health this fibrous skeleton forms approximately half the mass of the bloodless heart. In the normal subject the muscle mass amounts to approximately 250 g (Grande and Taylor, 1965). In arterial disease, because of the stress of an increased workload that is placed upon the circulation, the ratio of contractile to skeletal tissue may increase very substantially. The main coronary vessels lie in grooves of this skeleton where they are protected against the excesses of external compression by the heart muscle (Berne and Rubio, 1979).

All contractile tissue is capable of conducting electro-ionic impulses on its surface. Fibrous tissue does not possess this property (although in the trivial case it will conduct electrical charges when wetted with a salt-containing solution). Thus the only way that an ionic impulse can pass through the fibrous skeleton is via the atrio-ventricular bundle, a bundle of specialized conducting fibres. Impulses pass from the sinoatrial node in the right atrium down this bundle to the atrioventricular node and then on via the bundles of His which divide to straddle the interventricular septum, to pass directly to the apex of the ventricle and then reflect backwards, as the Purkinje fibres, towards the valvular rings across the base of the papillary muscles.

The functional arrangements of the muscle fibres of the ventricles are complex. Some muscle fibres form bundles which enclose both ventricles, others spiral around the individual ventricles, some form linear longitudinal bundles passing directly from the valvular ring to the apex, whilst yet others form figures of eight (Streeter, 1979). Although all muscle fibres are capable of conducting and propagating an impulse, the specialized conducting fibres within the heart conduct impulses at 2-4 m/s which is some ten times faster than the normal heart muscle fibre which conducts impulses at around 0·3 m/s (Milnor, 1980a). This has some significance when considering the propagation of an ectopic impulse.

The effect of all this arrangement on the functional efficiency of the ventricle is that the impulse for ventricular contraction reaches the apex of the heart, such that the apex contracts earlier and blood is being passed towards the outflow tract before the main body of the ventricular muscle is all fully depolarized. At this stage the cavity of the left ventricle assumes the shape of a ball until the aortic valve opens, whereas in the right ventricle the motion is more like a bellows (Parmley and Talbot, 1979). This arrangement in turn prevents undue mechanical stress or stretching on the apex of the heart (with the risk of herniation or aneurysmal deformations) before the aortic valve opens. When the apex of the ventricle is heavily scarred, as after previous apical myocardial infarction, the wave of contraction may not start at the apex but in the body of the ventricle. This imposes a very severe mechanical stress on the apex, depending upon the extent to which the apical contraction is out of phase with the contraction of the ventricular body, as blood within the apical portion of the cavity of the ventricle will not be able to escape very readily through the aortic valve. This predisposes to aneurysmal deformation of the ventricular wall. It is for this reason that apical aneurysms are so common among left ventricular aneurysms.

The septum between the two ventricles has a relatively thin muscle mass, so that if the ventricles contract asynchronously septal displacement would reduce the mechanical efficiency of the heart. In practice, particularly at slow heart rates, there is some degree of asynchronicity between the two ventricles but this is very minor. As the heart rate increases, or if there is increased sympathetic drive, the synchronicity improves and with it the mechanical efficiency of the heart (Brecher and Galletti, 1963).

The net effect of these structural and functional configurations is that the entire thrust of the ventricular contraction is directed against the aortic (or pulmonary) valve with the minimum of wasted effort. It is one of the fundamental principles of circulatory physiology that the heart works as hard as it has to and no more. The mechanism by which this is achieved is still not fully understood. In part, it is due to the specific properties of myocardial muscle and its contractility properties and in part to the controlling mechanisms of the vasomotor centre in the brain stem. How the brain stem recognizes when there is a need for an increase in cardiac output or change in heart rate is not known, yet the heart rate, stroke volume and blood pressure are meticulously controlled to ensure that there is the minimum of work by the heart for optimum flow to meet the total metabolic demands for oxygen and carbon dioxide transport. Both myocardial contractility and vasomotor centre control can be severely affected by anaesthesia, particularly control of heart rate which can materially affect the workload of the heart.

Probably the greatest single factor affecting the force, contractility and so functional efficiency of the ventricle is the end-diastolic pressure. Starling, many years ago (Starling, 1918), showed that a rise in the end-diastolic pressure provoked an augmented force of contraction of the next heart beat. Equally, if the ventricle is distended, so that the myocardial fibre length is increased, the same response occurs. The results of all these studies were the production of a family of Starling curves cross-relating end-diastolic pressure, myocardial fibre length and work done. These curves all have a similar form, a flattened parabola that is steep at the beginning, flattens out at high pressure ($20 \, cmH_2O$) and then descends at even higher pressures ($30 \, cmH_2O$) (Sarnoff, 1955). Subsequent work has shown that with chronic elevated pressures, as in chronic heart failure, there is some adaptation so that the level of pressure required before the curve flattens significantly becomes somewhat raised (Milnor, 1980b; Guyton, 1981a), but in these same subjects the margin of change in end-diastolic pressure between the curve flattening and the curve descending narrows. Clinically, patients in chronic heart failure may well have an end-diastolic pressure close to $20 \, cmH_2O$ and their hearts will respond to an increase in fluid load for an end-diastolic pressure of $25–35 \, cmH_2O$ but then fail abruptly with another small increment in load, i.e. their margin of reserve is much less.

Further work has extended the family of Starling curves. In the presence of catecholamines (Sarnoff, 1955) or a raised P_{CO_2} the curves are shifted to the Y-axis and become steeper, so that for a given end-diastolic pressure the work done is increased. Conversely if there is a metabolic acidosis the curves are flattened and depressed—the response is less and the descent occurs earlier and more quickly with further increases in end-diastolic pressure. With chronic acidosis, as in end-stage renal failure, this effect is less pronounced. Many drugs also do this, notably acetyl choline and its cogeners and the volatile anaesthetics at concentrations that would produce deep anaesthesia —although there is considerable variation between the different volatile agents (Etsten and Li, 1962). Deep halothane anaesthesia is the worst offender, whilst methoxyflurane is comparatively benign in this respect, with enflurane and isoflurane lying in between, although isoflurane is a worse offender than enflurane.

MYOCARDIAL CONTRACTILITY

From all this work has come the concept of 'myocardial contractility'. This term has many definitions—and indices: isometric tension index (Siegal and Sonnenblick, 1963); isotonic shortening (Noble et al., 1969); shortening velocity (Sonnenblick, 1965). Rushmer (1962) has propounded a general principle: that rates of change are significantly larger with changes in myocardial contractility than absolute changes of these units. This is reflected in the various indices of myocardial contractility that use a rate of change such as dP/dt_{max}—or the maximum rate of change of pressure within the ventricle before the aortic valve opens (Gleason and Braunwald, 1962); dQ/dt_{max}—or the maximum acceleration of the blood at the root of the aorta when the aortic valve opens and aortic impedance is at a minimum (Noble et al., 1969; Reitan et al., 1972). Other indices are time tension index (Sarnoff et al., 1958), cardiac output and so on. The simplest definition is the heart's ability to do work (Rusy, 1971). Cross-comparison of these various methods of evaluating myocardial contractility reveals good but not perfect agreement (Tomlin et al., 1975).

The reason for all these various indices is an attempt to give some quantitative indication of the heart's ability to do work, but this applies only to the work being done against the load or challenge offered within the physicochemical environment existing at the time of challenge. The clinician has a different viewpoint—he wishes to know not so much the heart's ability to do work (he can see that in front of him) but what reserve is there if the heart is called upon to work harder, or if the physicochemical environment should change? Can the patient's heart cope if there develops suddenly an episode of acidosis? Can the heart cope with an increased resistance load if the circulatory bed is suddenly reduced, as by the surgeon cross-clamping the descending aorta?

Preload

More commonly, the clinician wants to have some idea of the tolerance of response to changes in left ventricular end-diastolic pressure, which is related to, but is not synonymous with, changes in central venous pressure.

The key questions are:

> Does the patient need a high end-diastolic pressure or central venous pressure in order to generate an effective stroke volume and blood pressure?
>
> How will the heart cope with (a) a sudden decrease in venous return whether due to blood loss or the surgeon suddenly increasing the size of the vascular bed by releasing an important cross-clamp, or (b) an augmented venous return such as preloading with blood in anticipation of an expansion of the vascular bed by the surgeon?

After-load

Another significant factor in determining the work efficiency of the heart is the after-load (Sonnenblick and Downing, 1963), and this is particularly important in patients with degenerative vascular disease. In the normal heart with a stepwise increase in after-load or vascular resistance, it takes the heart 2–5 beats before it is once again expelling the same stroke volume and achieving the same end-diastolic pressure (Guyton, 1981b), yet the heart is manifestly working harder. It has to as the resistance against which it is working has increased. Initially, there is a transient reduction in stroke volume and an increase in end-diastolic pressure, but this quickly settles to normal levels. Originally, this response of increase in work output in response to an increase in vascular resistance was considered to be a consequence of an increased coronary perfusion resulting from the increase in arterial blood pressure. This explanation is wrong—even when the coronary vessels are being independently perfused at an unchanged pressure, this response to a change in after-load is seen (Berne, 1964). Conversely, when the resistance or after-load is diminished by inducing, by pharmacological means, vasodilatation or hypotension, the heart works less hard even if the coronary flow or pressure is deliberately augmented (Marchetti and Toccardi, 1967). The nerve fibres to the coronary vessels ensure that there is adequate coronary artery flow to meet any challenge given an adequate patency of the coronary vessels.

However, this situation is not true of the patient with occlusive arterial disease. If the coronary vessels are studded with atheroma, the coronary vasodilator fibres may be already working at their maximum. The whole coronary circulation becomes much more pressure-dependent. Two alternative situations may then arise: if there is hypotension for any reason the resulting arterial pressure may not be enough to ensure that all the necessary coronary flow can squeeze through the narrowed coronary vessels so that myocardial ischaemia and localized hypoxia occur, whilst, at its worst, stagnation of blood flow may develop which could precipitate thrombus formation and myocardial infarction. Alternatively, if there is an increase in vascular resistance, such as produced by cross-clamping the aorta, and therefore an extra work demand from the heart, the narrowed vessels may not allow all the increase in blood flow required to bring in the additional oxygen necessary for the increased metabolic activity for the additional work. Initially, there will be augmented extraction of what oxygen there is in the blood supplied, but if this is not enough local acidosis develops and this reduces local myocadial contractility. This throws further work on the rest of the heart muscle in its attempt to sustain the hypertension and a vicious spiral now develops leading to a rapidly rising end-diastolic pressure so that the heart moves to the inefficient part of the Starling curve and so develops acute heart failure. The subendocardial fibres are the most vulnerable in this respect (Guyton, 1981c). Thus, changes in after-load can disturb the normal coronary flow responses and with them myocardial contractility.

Potassium

Another factor affecting myocardial contractility is the level of intracellular potassium within the myocardial fibre. Within certain limits, the lower the intracellular potassium the greater is the contractility. During the depolarization phase of the cardiac cycle there is a considerable efflux of potassium from within the fibre to the extracellular fluid. The potassium has followed the concentration gradient as the depolarization has temporarily inhibited the system which constrains the potassium to within the cell. During repolarization, when the heart is in its refractory period, the sodium which had entered the cell during depolarization is now being actively extruded. Potassium has to re-enter the cell in order to maintain electrical balance of the positive ions. This process of sodium extrusion and potassium re-entry takes time. The potassium enters the cell in an exponential fashion, rapidly at first but with the process slowing as equilibrium is approached. The initial rate of entry is determined by the ratio of potassium concentration within the cell to that outside the cell. As the heart rate quickens so there is a reduction in the time available for that last portion of potassium to re-enter the cell. A new equilibrium of the ratio of potassium outside to inside the cell now develops. This means that the average (with respect to time) intracellular potassium falls slightly and this lowering of the intracellular potassium results in improved cardiac ejection (Van Winkle and Schwartz, 1976). With positive chronotropism there is thus a self-generating increase in myocardial contractility.

There is, however, a price to be paid. Intracellular potassium is needed to sustain a resting membrane potential. The nearer this potential is towards zero volts, the more easily it is triggered into an action potential (Hoffman and Cranefield, 1960). This trigger can be from any source, but this mechanism offers one explanation for why ectopic beats are more common during tachycardia. The converse, the appearance of ectopic beats during bradycardia, has a much more serious and sinister import. In this circumstance the instability of the membrane potential is not just an accidental by-product of the potassium balance, but is more likely due to a deranged enzyme system that is unable to achieve a proper ionic balance despite a long diastolic period. The commonest cause for this is tissue hypoxia, due either to ischaemia or to hypoxaemia.

SOME EFFECTS OF DEGENERATIVE VASCULAR DISEASE ON THE FUNCTIONAL EFFICIENCY OF THE HEART

In degenerative vascular disease this complex arrangement may be severely disturbed, depending upon the pattern of this disease. Patches of atheroma may lead to ischaemic degeneration of the atrioventricular bundle, so causing complete heart block with the atrioventricular node acting as the pacemaker. The normal pacemaker is the sino-atrial node which has a natural slow frequency, but this frequency is considerably modified by the balance of neuronal discharges reaching it either from the sympathetic system (which increases the frequency) of from the parasympathetic system (which decreases the frequency). These neuronal discharges in turn may be reflex in origin or arise from the vasomotor centre in the brain stem. In contrast the atrioventricular node has little functional neuronal input (Thaemert, 1970). Left to itself it would discharge at a slow frequency of 30–50 beats per minute, a frequency which is suboptimal as far as work done is concerned. Hence degenerative heart disease affecting the atrioventricular bundle that induces complete heart block causes considerable heart slowing. This, with an unchanged venous return, must mean that stroke volume must increase from its normal value of 70 ml per beat to as much as 140 ml per beat, which necessitates a very distended ventricular chamber and this in turn has a knock-on effect on the myocardial efficiency via the Starling mechanism.

A different effect that degenerative vascular disease may have on the heart is ischaemic failure of one of the conducting bundles, causing either right or left bundle branch block. This in turn causes some asynchronicity in ventricular contraction and hence reduced mechanical efficiency. This disturbance in the timing relationships may be seen on the ECG. Of itself this reduction in myocardial efficiency is relatively minor unless, for other reasons, the heart needs to be at maximum mechanical efficiency for what little blood or oxygen supply it may be receiving.

Ectopic beats

A not infrequent feature of degenerative vascular disease is a patch of coronary atheroma leading to a small scar on the ventricular wall. This may be of full or partial thickness. This scar is the scavenged remnant of a small zone of infarction (which could have been clinically silent). At the margins of the scar are zones of muscle with a reduced blood supply, not so reduced that the fibres die but reduced so that survival of these fibres is precarious. The fibres do work when contracting. Some of this work is mechanical work, but some is biochemical. Energy is required to expel the sodium ions that enter the fibres during depolarization, the so-called 'sodium pump'. Energy is also required to maintain the resting membrane potential during diastole. The nearer the resting membrane potential approaches zero volts (Trautwein, 1963), the more easily it may be provoked into an action potential. A deficit in the local oxygen supply will make the achievement of a stable resting membrane potential that much more difficult. Any other factor which causes instability of the resting membrane potential (and this might be an increase in catecholamines, a raised $Paco_2$ or the presence of a volatile anaesthetic, or any combination of these) will interact initially with such a zone of instability. This unstable focus then triggers into an action potential. The resulting impulse is propagated across the heart muscle directly passing from fibre to fibre, sweeping across the heart uniformly.

The aberrant impulse propagates at a rate that is ten times slower than the rate that normal impulses are conducted down the bundles of His (Milnor, 1980a). This slowness is reflected in the widening of the would-be QRS complex of the ectopic wave of depolarization. As a result of this slow wave of depolarization, some parts of the heart depolarize and contract whilst other parts of the heart are still awaiting the arrival of the aberrant impulse. Ventricular contraction is therefore highly asynchronous and little effective work or cardiac ejection is done. As some parts of the ventricular wall contract, they dimple the blood within the chamber which is reflected as a slight distension of the remainder of the relaxed ventricular wall. This is the phenomenon of the ectopic beat. Another consequence of an ectopic beat is the time factor. During the propagation of an ectopic beat the muscle fibres depolarize. Then they must repolarize, but this takes time. Meanwhile the venous return continues unabated and the ventricle distends. The next heart beat will have an augmented stroke volume and stroke pressure via the Starling mechanism and little harm is done.

This is not the case if there are multiple foci of ectopic impulses or runs of ectopics from a single focus, as these may lead to repetitive over-stretching of the ventricle and eventually lead to heart failure. More importantly, they may presage the onset of ventricular fibrillation.

In chronic degenerative vascular disease where there has been much ventricular hypertrophy consequent upon associated hypertension, the subendocardial fibres are placed at a distinct disadvantage (Guyton, 1981c). As a result of the ventricular hypertrophy, the distance the coronary blood has to travel during diastole to reach the subendocardial areas is increased, as blood flows from the exterior towards the interior of the heart. This flow only occurs in diastole as during systole the smaller intramural vessels are compressed and their contents squeezed out. Because of the hypertension the myocardial fibres are also working harder. The extraction of oxygen at the subendocardial zone is then maximal and yet the mean oxygen tension of this zone may be very low, much lower than in the main part of the heart muscle. These subendocardial fibres of the hypertrophied ventricle are particularly vulnerable to hypoxaemia (Guyton, 1981c), hypercapnia and halogenated hydrocarbons. If the ventricle is then stressed, by a sudden attempt to increase myocardial contractility such as to meet an increase in after-load, the subendocardial fibres may not receive enough oxygen relative to their metabolic demand. Their ability to re-establish and maintain a stable resting membrane potential after a wave of contraction may be sufficiently impaired that they will act as a focus for an ectopic wave of depolarization. Thus ectopic beats are not always just due to previous scarring of the heart muscle.

BLOOD FLOW IN THE RIGHT VENTRICLE

Blood enters the right atrium through the superior and inferior venae cavae and the coronary sinus. The venous oxygen tension of blood from each of these sources is quite different. At rest the blood in the inferior vena cava has a high oxygen content because much of the blood flowing through this vein has gone through tissues for purposes other than meeting simple local metabolic demand, e.g. the kidney has a blood flow that is very substantially in excess of its metabolic needs, hence renal vein blood has a high oxygen content. In contrast, coronary sinus blood is particularly low in oxygen since it has to meet the oxygen debt incurred during systole. On average, coronary sinus blood has suffered a 50% extraction of its oxygen (Gregg and Fisher, 1963) but in the hard-working, hypertrophied, hypertensive heart the oxygen extraction is considerably higher (hence this explains why patients with hypertension and coronary atherosclerosis withstand hypoxia or a reduction in available coronary oxygen supply so badly). These differing oxygen concentrations in different streams of blood within the right atrium make right atrial blood valueless for cardiac output estimations using the Fick method. Similarly, right atrial blood is also useless in attempts to quantify arteriovenous shunting in the peripheral circulation (such shunting occurs in some forms of shock, in heat conservation when the patient is exposed to hypothermic conditions, and in arteriovenous fistulas whether natural or artificial).

The blood enters the right ventricle at an angle to the atrial inflows and this favours the continuation of the streaming. *In utero* this streaming principle is particularly important in optimizing oxygenation of the developing brain. In adults during systole there is considerable mixing of these various streams but the mixing is by no means complete. Even after ejection through the pulmonary valve and the turbulent mixing that occurs there as the blood enters the pulmonary artery, the mixing is still not quite complete. Blood entering the right pulmonary artery and destined for the right lung has a slightly greater proportion of superior vena caval blood than blood in the left pulmonary artery (Brecher and Galletti, 1963). This difference is only a matter of a few per cent but it does bring into question the precision of cardiac output determinations using the thermal dilution technique (in which it is assumed that complete mixing and thermal equilibration occur within the right ventricle and also that there is no heat or cold exchange between the blood and the ventricular wall).

There is one other aid to mechanical efficiency within the right ventricle. Because of the angular arrangements of the venous inflow the blood flows in a markedly ellipsoid fashion, i.e. it does not enter, come to a complete stop and then reverse its direction of movement with all the loss of inertial energy that this implies. Because of this ellipsoid path some of the blood maintains its momentum and is 'whipped on' by the bellows-like contraction of the right ventricle towards the ventricular outflow tract. In degenerative vascular disease, particularly if there is any pulmonary hypertension consequent upon left ventricular failure, the isovolumetric phase of ventricular contraction may be prolonged whilst the ventricle builds up its pressure to overcome the raised pulmonary vascular resistance. This means that the blood movement has to stop and then start to move again; that is, there is some loss of the conservation of momentum.

THE CARDIAC CYCLE

The peak of the P wave of the ECG, or electrocardiograph, marks the start of the physical contraction of the atrium and the start of the 'a' wave of the jugular venous wave. The ventricle is quiescent in protosystole, while the electrical impulse continues its passage through the a–v node and down the bundles of His. This initiates ventricular systole.

Mechanical systole starts at the height of the R wave (Brecher and Galletti, 1963). During the first part, the period of isovolumetric contraction, the ventricle changes shape, as the apex contracts first and the intraventricular pressure rises. This causes the cavity of the left ventricle to become ball-shaped, but the right ventricular cavity is bellows-shaped. In this first part of ventricular systole the aortic valve is closed and remains so until the S wave of the ECG is completed.

Inotropism

Inotropism appertains to alterations in myocardial contractility. Anything that increases the myocardial contractility is said to exhibit positive inotropism, whilst anything that lowers myocardial contractility is said to show negative inotropism. This term 'myocardial contractility' is an elusive one for which many definitions have been made, all slightly differing from each other depending upon the method of assessing myocardial contractility. The consensus definition of myocardial contractility is the ability to do work (Rusy, 1971), which obviously cannot be tested until the work is actually undertaken. One of the many definitions of myocardial contractility is the maximum rate of change of pressure, dP/dt_{max} (Gleason and Braunwald, 1962). This can only be measured experimentally by having a catheter placed within the ventricle connected by a very short rigid tube to a transducer (or, alternatively, a transducer-tipped catheter probe), so that there is minimum distortion of the transduced pressure signal (Gersch et al., 1971; Prys-Roberts et al., 1972). This signal is then instantly differentiated to identify the rate of change of pressure with time and then the maximum of this is measured. Electronically this is done by analogue differentiation, that is, obtaining the differential of the change of pressure with respect to time and then plotting this differential against time on a pen recorder. The peak height of the differential trace is the maximum rate of change of pressure with time. An analogue of the concept of dP/dt_{max} is peak acceleration or the maximum rate of change of velocity, dV/dt_{max}, during cardiac ejection, although in time this occurs after dP/dt_{max} (which by definition occurs during the isovolumetric phase which is prior to the opening of the aortic valve).

During catecholamine stimulation or a sympathetic nervous system discharge (or the use of certain sympathomimetic agents), there is an increase in myocardial contractility. The maximum rate of change of pressure is reached earlier during the isovolumetric contraction phase. This is sometimes called a 'positive inotropism'. Inotropism should not be confused with chronotropism which relates to changes in the heart rate. If a drug or sympathetic stimulation causes the heart rate to increase this is positive chronotropism. Usually inotropism and chronotropism go hand in hand, but there are exceptions; thus calcium ions have a powerful positive inotropic effect but little to no chronotropic effect.

Negative inotropism is the reverse. The maximum rate of the change of pressure is less and occurs later in the isovolumetric contraction phase. The heart has a reduced ability to do work whilst under the effect of negative inotropic influences. Such influences are parasympathetic nervous system stimulation (which also slows the heart), or vagal stimulation, or light halothane anaesthesia. If these negative inotropic influences are not too powerful, the final systolic pressure may remain unchanged. Only the heart muscle is contracting sluggishly and if challenged, e.g. by cross-clamping the aorta, the heart muscle may not be able to respond to the increased resistance load and under these circumstances cardiac output may not be sustained. Negative inotropism is not normally a clinical problem, unless there is negative chronotropism, the one exception being the effects of short acting barbiturate induction agents, when left ventricular end-diastolic pressure, left atrial pressure and pulmonary artery wedge pressure all may rise sharply but the heart rate remains undisturbed (Price and Dripps, 1971).

The patient with major peripheral vascular disease often has associated hypertension. With the increase in diastolic blood pressure of hypertension the period of isovolumetric contraction may be lengthened slightly. dP/dt_{max} is attained early in the period of isovolumetric contraction and then sustained at this rate until the intraventricular pressure causes the aortic valve to open. The ventricle is working much harder and is nearer to its failing limit.

A second effect that is commonly seen in the elderly patient with degenerative vascular disease is that, in response to a painful stimulus, instead of the normal sympathetic discharge the response is a parasympathetic one, with a marked bradycardia, a depression in myocardial contractility and a marked lowering of the systolic blood pressure. This is usually accompanied by a fall in cardiac output.

The next phase of the cardiac cycle is the rapid ejection phase. In time this occurs from the middle to end of the S wave until halfway through the T wave of the ECG. In this phase both mitral and tricuspid valves are shut tight and the atrial and central venous pressure starts to rise. This corresponds to the ascending part of the v wave on the venous pressure wave complex.

The rate of ejection depends upon the myocardial contractility and the impedance of the aorta. Thus for any one patient the rate of change of flow or the acceleration of blood flow at the root of the aorta is also a measure of myocardial contractility. Intravascular electromagnetic flow probes have been used in man, experimentally (Mills and Shillingford, 1967) for this assessment. In the fit, healthy subject this impedance is low (Gersh et al., 1972). The normal aorta is very elastic and distends readily under pressure as the rate of ejection is usually faster than blood can flow down the aorta. During diastole, the distended aorta recoils as the pressure dies away and that blood which has been stored in this distension is then discharged down the aorta to the periphery (*Fig.* 1.1). This is the diastolic pump and it accounts for between 25–40% of the stroke volume. One important effect of the diastolic pump is that the average velocity of blood flowing down the aorta is lessened by this effect. Since the energy demand is a function of the square of the velocity this diastolic pump effect, due to aortic distensibility, makes a considerable saving of energy. The energy required to push the blood through the aorta is reduced to only 7% of what it would be if the aorta were a rigid tube of the diameter of the normal aorta (O'Rourke, 1967). This uncoupling effect of the elasticity of the aorta is thus a great energy saver and spares the heart much work.

In the patients with degenerative vascular disease there is considerable loss of elastic tissue, particulary at the aortic arch and thoracic aorta as well as at major bifurcations or origins of the principal arteries. As a result of being subject to mechanical distending forces of every heart beat the degenerating aorta slowly distends and stretches and dilates, causing the aortic knuckle to unfold somewhat. Nevertheless, the aortic impedance has risen sharply and the heart has to work harder to overcome this. The diastolic pump is also less effective and the net result is that much more of the stroke volume has to be delivered to the peripheral tissues during systole. This markedly increases the velocity of blood during systole which produces another effect. The Reynolds number is a dimensionless entity which is related to the velocity of flow of a liquid through a tube (named after Osborne Reynolds, it is the product of the velocity of flow, diameter of the tube and density of the liquid divided by the viscosity of that liquid; Uvarov et al., 1973). At a certain critical value it heralds the appearance of turbulent flow. Since the diameter, density and viscosity are all relatively constant, this critical value corresponds to a critical velocity. The critical Reynolds number is exceeded in the ascending aorta and aortic arch—so that there is considerable turbulence there. In the descending thoracic aorta in the normal subject the flow

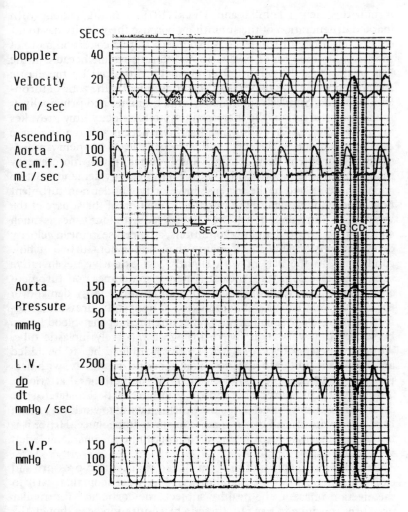

Fig. 1.1.   **The inter-relationship of events in the cardiac cycle.**
  A. **Start of systole. Left ventricular pressure starts to rise.**
  B. **Electromagnetic flow (e.m.f.) probe on the ascending aorta shows opening of aortic valve and the start of flow in the aorta.**
  C. **Closure of aortic valve. Aortic inflow has ceased but the Doppler probe on the descending aorta still shows forward flow.**
  D. **Elastic recoil and the diastolic pump effect starting at the dichrotic notch. The stippled area is diastolic flow.**

(Reproduced with acknowledgements from Tomlin P. J. and Duck F. A. (1974) Total peripheral resistance and diastolic blood flow. *Can. Anaesth. Soc. J.* **21**: 482.)

is non-turbulent (Tomlin and Duck, 1975). In the patient with marked degeneration of the subintima, because the velocity has to increase, the zone of turbulence is extended. In this condition more of the stroke volume has to be distributed during systole because of the loss of the diastolic pump effect normally produced by the elastic aorta. Hence flow has to be faster and consequently the zone of turbulence extends. Similarly, at major arterial branches and principally at the aortic bifurcation, the increase in systolic velocity now provokes more turbulence. The turbulence itself also acts as a distending force causing dilatation of the aorta and eventually leads to aneurysm formation. Turbulent flow demands (and wastes) much more energy than non-turbulent flow (Hill, 1980). To this energy demand must be added those related to the increase in velocity—under non-turbulent flow conditions the energy required is a function of the square of the velocity, so that a doubling of the velocity requires four times as much energy. Under turbulent flow conditions, an increase in mean velocity demands considerably more energy than under non-turbulent flow conditions. In the patient with slightly less extensive degenerative subintimal disease, within the aorta, flow is sometimes non-turbulent and sometimes turbulent, but the instantaneous energy demand of the heart is very considerably increased. The systolic pressure therefore increases very substantially, reflecting the fact that blood has to be squeezed at very high speed through a relatively inelastic tube. The heart is working very hard. To this workload has to be added another factor. Often there is some more peripheral disease with narrowing of and possible loss of elasticity at the peripheral arterioles. The diastolic pressure, which more readily reflects the state of the arterioles, therefore rises. Thus the heart is having to work very much harder to overcome all these changes in aortic impedance. Hence it is not surprising that often in these patients there is considerable left ventricular hypertrophy.

Oscilloscopic displays of the transduced signals from pressure and electromagnetic flow probes at the ascending aorta show that, early in the ejection phase in the healthy subject, the aortic and ventricular pressures continue to rise rapidly for a brief duration even though the blood is flowing from the ventricle and down the aorta. There is an initial spike of pressure and flow which rapidly settles to a plateau where the pressure and flow signals, e.g. thoracic aortic flow, are almost indistinguishable (Spencer and Dennison, 1963). Pressure signals, acquired via transducers used for sensing pressures further downstream, do not show this pattern in the young healthy subject; the elasticity of the aorta and of the arterial tree dampen down the near rectangular pressure wave to produce a rounded hump of pressure. In contrast, in the patient with major arterial disease with a significant loss of the subintimal elasticity, the pattern, during systole, of the pressure signal obtained from a transducer and displayed on an oscilloscope is more usually preserved, even when the signal is acquired at the level of the radial artery. That is to say, in patients with arterial disease, the radial artery pressure wave in the first part of systole reflects the situation at the root of the aorta.

More significantly, if this pattern is seen in a patient and then during anaesthesia it should change, this reflects an alteration in the haemodynamics of the rapid ejection phase of the cardiac cycle. If there is a failure in sustaining the plateau of pressure in the first part of systole, this may mean that the ventricle is not sustaining its normal ejection pattern: either the venous return is inadequate and the heart has not enough blood to eject, or else myocardial contractility is failing. If it is the latter, the upstroke of the radial artery pressure signal is sluggish (even though it retains its other features such as the dichrotic notches which would otherwise indicate that this degradation of signal is artefactual). If the heart is healthy and it is a matter of a failing venous return, the upstroke of the pressure wave is normal, sharp, crisp and quick. This sign, of a failing to maintain a plateau of pressure that was previously seen, is one of the earliest indicators of a significant disruption of the circulatory haemodynamics, the most vulnerable and most easily disturbed being the rapid ejection phase of the cardiac cycle.

SYMPATHETIC AND PARASYMPATHETIC DRIVE

A certain amount of sympathetic nervous drive, either directly through the sympathetic nervous system or indirectly through the catecholamine secretions of the adrenal medulla, are necessary for sustained cardiac effort. Total failure of the sympathetic nervous system, or vasomotor centre paralysis, induces widespread vasodilatation. The venous return falls and the heart is unable to respond, so the blood pressure falls. The normal response to hypotension is the baroreceptor response (Little, 1981a). Stretch receptors, mainly in the aortic arch but also present at the origins of all the major vessels opening from the aorta, sense this hypotension. Stimuli are sent to the vasomotor centre whose response is a sympathetic arousal inducing, particularly, tachycardia. There is also pulmonary vasoconstriction. Within the pulmonary vascular bed there is a reserve of 300–600 ml of blood (Keele et al., 1982a). Pulmonary vasoconstriction thus augments the venous return to the left ventricle. The pulmonary vasoconstriction, in turn, causes the ventricle to be suddenly stretched and this, in turn, induces an increase in contractility. The increased left ventricular output, hopefully, improves the blood pressure until such time as the systemic venous return has increased to take over. The beneficial effects of this are much less during controlled ventilation because of the Valsalva (Valsalva, 1704; Dawson, 1943) effects of positive pressure ventilation. Total failure of the sympathetic nervous system results in a progressive diminution of cardiac output and with it hypotension, causing a reduced and eventual failure of the coronary perfusion with cardiac anoxia and death of the heart. Such a situation occurs in brain-stem death and takes a few days to develop (Jennet et al., 1981). If there is any reduction in adrenal medullary secretion this process is accelerated.

The overall effects of sympathetic stimulation are:

1. The ventricular function curve is moved towards the Y axis so that the heart produces more work for any given ventricular end-diastolic pressure or length (stretching) of the myocardial muscle fibres.
2. The relationship between end-diastolic pressure and fibre length is preserved unchanged—that is, the heart is just as stretchable.
3. There is improved ejection of the blood from the ventricle as a result of the increase in contractility, so that the end-diastolic pressure falls until the venous return increases consequent upon the improved cardiac output.
4. Systole is shortened relative to diastole, so that per minute there is increased time to fill the ventricles.
5. Diastole is also shortened per heart beat thereby increasing the overall heart rate—positive chronotropism.
6. The myocardial contractility is increased further by virtue of reducing the time at each heart beat for the potassium to re-enter the fibres so that intracellular potassium falls.
7. By increasing the heart rate, the synchronicity of contraction of all the heart muscle fibres is improved, thereby increasing the mechanical efficiency of the heart. (The reverse is total asynchronicity of contraction as in ventricular fibrillation when no effective work is done.)
8. There is an increase in the rate of propagation of impulses through the whole conducting system within the heart, so that not only is conduction between and through the atrioventricular node quickened—thereby shortening the P–R interval of the ECG—but also there is an increase in the velocity of propagation or spread of the wave of depolarization, so that the QRS time is also shortened. This, in turn, aids the synchronicity of contraction of all the myocardial fibres.

Parasympathetic stimulation has precisely the opposite effects. In particular, it causes very marked bradycardia up to and including asystole. In the healthy heart, after a period of 4–30 s there is then the phenomenon of vagal escape. The sinoatrial node has its own natural rhythm and it will start to produce its own regular signals. These will be propagated in the usual way and so regular rhythmical heart beats will occur. This will restart the coronary perfusion and any acetylcholine left at the sinoatrial node will be washed away. Repetitive doses of succinylcholine will have the same effect (Bullough, 1959; Tomlin and Duck, 1975). During the period of asystole, the venous return to both ventricles, from the pulmonary and systemic circulations, will still continue and the respective ventricles will become distended with an increase in their relative end-diastolic pressures. The first one or two heart beats will be augmented via the Starling mechanism, but thereafter stroke volume and heart rate will resume their normal dimensions. If the heart is being exposed to some toxic process, e.g. after a burns injury, septicaemia or toxaemia, vagal escape is much less likely. In the patient with atherosclerosis there may well be a zone of myocardial ischaemia with a patch of myocardial tissue that has an unstable resting membrane potential. As a result of the further tissue hypoxia consequent upon the cardiac standstill, this patch may then become a focus for ectopic beats. Since the ectopic beats are mechanically very ineffective there is little to no coronary perfusion, so that any residual oxygen left in the heart tissue is rapidly consumed. The heart may then pass straight from asystole to ventricular fibrillation.

Sympathetic nervous system stimulation is enhanced by some anaesthetic agents, notably ether and cyclopropane (Price et al., 1967; Marshall and Wollman, 1980) and is diminished by others such as halothane (Skovsted et al., 1972). Hypercapnia increases the sympathetic drive, although this effect is largely obtunded during anaesthesia, the final result depending upon the choice of anaesthetic drug. Hypocapnia has the reverse effect. Pain in young subjects normally provokes a sympathetic response, although in the old it not infrequently produces a parasympathetic response. A metabolic acidosis blocks the effects of sympathetic stimulation on the heart, the extent of the block depending upon the extent of the acidosis.

Hypoxia produces a biphasic response. Initially, there is augmentation of sympathetic activity with a marked increase in cardiac output and arterial blood pressure (to the point of petechial haemorrhages on the surface of the brain and pericardium). There is also an initial tachycardia but, as the hypoxia is prolonged, the parasympathetic system takes over with a marked bradycardia and hypotension. There is a progressive fall of contractility until only slow, bizarre ECG complexes can be obtained with no muscle contraction or cardiac ejection. Then ventricular fibrillation occurs. A few people respond idiosynchratically to hypoxia by moving directly to the parasympathetic–bradycardiac response. In the elderly patient with severe occlusive arterial disease the sympathetic response to hypoxia is very much less marked.

THE EFFECTS OF pH, CALCIUM IONS, P_{O_2}, P_{CO_2}

pH effects

Substrate utilization and energy production are the result of the actions of a multiplicity of intracellular enzymatic processes. These enzymes operate over a narrow range of hydrogen ion concentration and a progressive departure from the optimum results in less and less enzymatic efficiency. This is an exponential process related to the reciprocal of the hydrogen ion concentration. As far as the heart is concerned, at a constant P_{CO_2} there is a linear relationship between the logarithm of the reciprocal of the hydrogen ion concentration (or pH) and the cardiac output (converting the hydrogen ion concentration into a logarithmic notation converts the exponential format into a linear one). At an arterial pH of 7·40 or 40 nmol hydrogen ion concentration, the cardiac output is maximal for the minimum cardiac work relative to metabolic needs. At a pH of 7·15 or 83 nmol hydrogen ion concentration, the cardiac output is half of what it should be (Tomlin, 1966), whilst at a pH of 6·90 or 120 nmol hydrogen ion concentration, cardiac output is virtually zero, all at normal P_{CO_2} levels. In the newborn these limits are extended somewhat, but even in the newborn a pH of 6·75 or 150 nmol hydrogen ion concentration is incompatible with survival. In the patient with degenerative arterial disease, in which there is a crucial need to sustain a good ejection pressure to compensate for the loss of aortic elasticity, the fall in myocardial contractility consequent upon metabolic acidosis results in a precipitate fall in systolic blood pressure to half or less of what is necessary, with all the consequent hazards as far as the renal or coronary perfusions are concerned.

Calcium ions

Inter-related to the pH is the level of ionized calcium. Calcium ions are essential for the coupling process of the myoglobin molecules. In this process myosin, a long 1000 Ångström units molecule, couples with actin to form actinomyosin and in the presence of calcium ions the molecule folds dramatically. Little energy is needed for this folding to take place but considerable energy is needed to sustain it.

If the level of ionized calcium falls, myocardial contractility falls and with it both cardiac output and peak ejection pressure fall. In clinical anaesthesia this is rarely a problem except under two specific situations. (a) The first is an inability to remove effectively the citrate in transfused blood. The principal organ for the removal of citrate is the liver and at normothermia the healthy liver can deal with all the citrate in 1 unit of blood in 3 min. Hence any transfusion in which blood is transfused at a rate slower than 1 unit per 3 min at normothermia is unlikely to precipitate citrate intoxication or a depletion in the level of ionized calcium. In hypothermia this 3 min period is extended significantly, the magnitude of the extension being dependent upon the degree of hypothermia—but even a fall in body core temperature of only 2 or 3 °C can have a significant effect clinically. After large blood transfusions it may take the liver a little longer to cope, i.e., up to 6 min per unit of blood. Large volume transfusions, 10 units of blood or more, are an occasional feature in the clinical management of patients undergoing major vascular surgery. At the extreme, large falls in ionized calcium are seen during the anhepatic phase of a liver transplant operation (Gray et al., 1985), but even during major surgery on the lower aorta should the patient become hypothermic (and this is common) depletion of ionized calcium is a significant hazard if blood has to be transfused quickly. (b) The second specific situation in which there may be a precipitous fall in the level of ionized calcium is when a metabolic acidosis is reversed too abruptly by a sodium bicarbonate infusion. Calcium ions react with bicarbonate to form a chalky precipitate which does nothing for the acidosis. It is therefore necessary to give the bicarbonate in slow increments to allow for the physical buffering of the bicarbonate by the serum albumin and for the mobilization of calcium ions by the liver, otherwise the fall in myocardial contractility consequent upon the acidosis is then replaced by a fall in myocardial contractility consequent upon a fall in the level of ionized calcium.

Pa_{CO_2} Changes in Pa_{CO_2} affect the circulation in four ways.

1. As a result of an increase in intracranial Pa_{CO_2}, there is increased activity of the vasomotor centre, resulting in an increased discharge to the heart via the cardiac sympathetic nerves.
2. There is also an increased production of adrenaline from the adrenal medulla, and this significantly affects myocardial performance.
3. An increase in carbon dioxide tension causes an increase in the serum potassium level; there is a linear relationship between the two (Hassan et al., 1979). The increase in potassium is due to an increase in the intracellular positive ions resulting from the respiratory acidosis. Since potassium re-enters the cell passively to maintain ionic balance after muscle fibre depolarization and subsequent ionic sodium extrusion, the increase in intracellular hydrogen ions acts as a brake. This, in turn, increases myocardial contractility and with it myocardial irritability, as has been discussed earlier in this chapter (page 7).
4. Carbon dioxide directly increases myocardial contractility and

irritability in its own right, even when the hydrogen ion change consequent upon the respiratory acidosis is neutralized.

There is considerable species difference, the irritability being very considerably less in the dog (which makes transfer to man of experimental results obtained from the dog where they involve changes in carbon dioxide tension and the circulation slightly suspect, and explains the success of the first ever inhalational anaesthetic (Smith, 1978) that was given by Henry Hill Hickman to his dog). The combination of a raised Pa_{CO_2}, an increased production of endogenous adrenaline and the presence of certain anaesthetic vapours poses a particular threat of multifocal ventricular extrasystoles and even ventricular fibrillation. Given enough of each, each will do it in its own right but the three do synergize with each other. Different anaesthetic vapours do each have a particular level of Pa_{CO_2} at which arrhythmias are precipitated at the same effective anaesthetic concentration (MAC1, or minimum alveolar concentration to produce light surgical anaesthesia) (Raftery, 1980) and these arrhythmias can be blocked by beta-blocking drugs. If, however, the patient has an irritable focus, a zone of heart muscle where the resting membrane potential is less stable than normal as a result, say, of chronic ischaemia, the arrhythmia will develop at a Pa_{CO_2} level that would be considered as being below the arrhythmic threshold. This situation is particularly apposite for the patient undergoing anaesthesia for vascular surgery. Even though the patient has no overt signs or symptoms of ischaemic heart disease, nor any ECG evidence of ischaemia, nevertheless the risk of developing abnormal heart beats if there is any carbon dioxide retention is much higher in these patients, the patients at particular risk being those suffering from hypertension.

Respiratory acidosis offsets the depression in myocardial contractility produced by the change of hydrogen ion concentration. There may even be an increase in cardiac output but the extent of this will depend upon the background anaesthetic agent. In the dog the response, of an increase in cardiac output, is much greater for the same degree of respiratory acidosis with a barbiturate type of anaesthesia than with light halothane anaesthesia (Carson et al., 1965; Tomlin, 1966).

Hypoxia

The hardest-working portion of the heart is the left ventricle. Over 90% of the blood flow of the left ventricle wall passes through the coronary sinus as there are few thebesian veins in the left ventricular wall (William and Warwick, 1980). At rest, in normal subjects, the coronary sinus blood is only 35% saturated with oxygen (Little,

1981b) as compared with 75% saturated for the average venous return. That is, whilst the rest of the body consumes only one-quarter of the oxygen with which it is supplied and so has a reasonable reserve to tolerate any reduction in supply, the left ventricle consumes half of what it is supplied with, so that its tolerance to a reduction in supply is reduced. The effect of hypoxia on the heart will depend upon the heart's previous history. The energy required for myocardial contraction is mainly supplied by the oxidation of fat (60%) via the Krebs citric acid cycle (Ganong, 1983a). The source of free fatty acid is that in the arterial blood. In addition, the heart can metabolize amino acids (5%) and carbohydrate (35%). The heart also has a limited supply of glycogen stored in its fibres. A low blood sugar would adversely affect myocardial contractility if it were not for the sympathetic response to hypoglycaemia. This response is partially blocked by anaesthesia.

Theoretically, a hypertensive diabetic patient whose current medication includes beta-blocking drugs and who becomes severely hypoglycaemic is at risk. In practice, although hypertensive diabetics are commonly found among patients undergoing vascular surgery, their form of diabetes is such that the patient is unlikely to become severely hypoglycaemic unless there has been some clinical error. Faced with a shortage of energy, the heart will utilize what anaerobic means of metabolism it can, mainly keto-oxidation and using what glycogen it has in store. The latter will be metabolized as far as pyruvic and then lactic acid. Eventually the acidosis predominates and this depresses the myocardial contractility. If the recent medical history is one of a severe catabolic stress—whether by septicaemia, burst abdomen or renal failure—this glycogen reserve is depleted and the tolerance to hypoxia is much reduced.

During myocardial contraction the myoglobin molecules fold. Although little energy is needed to initiate the coupling and folding process, a lot of energy is needed to sustain the physical configuration of these molecules. This is reflected in the way the heart beats when there is severe hypoxia—when contractions become snatched and short lived between progressively increasing periods of diastole.

Apart from the effects on the sympathetic system previously described, lesser degrees of hypoxia provoke a marked increase in coronary artery dilatation (Schlant et al., 1982). The coronary vessels have the capacity of increasing coronary artery blood flow up to five times normal (Berne, 1964), but in the atherosclerotic patient this reserve capacity is much less. Indeed, coronary vessel dilatation may be the maximum possible so that there is no reserve. Under these conditions the coronary blood flow, and thereby the degree of coronary oxygenation become entirely pressure dependent. The extraction of oxygen from the arterial blood increases at all levels of heart muscle and there is a marked autoregulatory mechanism to divert blood to areas of localized severe hypoxia (Schlant et al., 1982). Nevertheless, the subendocardial layers are extracting all the oxygen from the blood supply that they can and the oxygen tension of the emerging end capillary blood will be approaching zero.

Clinically, the effects of hypoxia are a mass sympathetic stimulation and a positive inotropic effect on the heart, the duration of which will depend upon the previous state of health of the heart. Then it passes to a negative inotropic response and negative chronotropism, leading to bradycardia and then ventricular fibrillation, but if the energy reserve has been seriously depleted asystole will occur rather than ventricular fibrillation.

ELECTROPHYSIOLOGICAL CONSIDERATIONS

Detailed consideration of the various ECG changes that may be seen in patients undergoing vascular surgery is beyond the scope of this book. They do reflect the whole gamut of the ECG changes of ischaemic heart disease; left, right or both left and right ventricular hypertrophy, total heart block, bundle branch block, left or right axis deviation and so on. There are, however, one or two aspects of the ECG which are of particular interest to the anaesthetist.

The first of these is related to timing of the various physiological events of the cardiac cycle. First there is the P wave, which corresponds to atrial depolarization. Then there is the P–R interval, which reflects the velocity of propagation of an impulse through the conducting system of the heart. The fact that the velocity of propagation is responsive to the level of sympathetic activity changes in the P–R interval, particularly if it is shortening, can provide another indicator that whatever stimulus is being applied it is evoking a sympathetic response. Since a number of anaesthetic techniques coincidentally cause some suppression of other responses of the sympathetic nervous system, this can be a useful indicator. The ideal lead to obtain the maximum size of the P wave and P–R interval is lead 2 of the ECG.

The next wave following the P wave is the QRS complex. This marks the spread of the wave of depolarization. Ischaemic areas will deform the QRS complex, whilst bundle branch block causes marked notching of the complex. Changes in the QRS profile during anaesthesia in patients with vascular disease may indicate that some parts of the heart are hypoxic. It is, however, an unreliable and very late (by anaesthetic standards) sign. The wave of electrical depolarization is synchronous with the wave of mechanical ventricular contraction —and this then provides a useful indicator of the velocity of propagation of either a flow or pressure wave to the peripheral arteries. For example, if a flow detector is placed over the thumb and its electrical output displayed on the same oscilloscope on which is displayed the ECG, the interval between the QRS complex and the flow wave signal reflects the time from ventricular contraction to the flow resulting from that contraction actually arriving at the thumb. If this time interval increases, this means that the velocity of flow has reduced, that is, ventricular ejection velocity has deteriorated—and this, in turn, means that myocardial contractility has deteriorated.

The T wave reflects repolarization. Since depolarization and repolarization are independent of each other, the path of the T wave does not follow the path of the QRS wave (Milnor, 1980c). Repolarization starts from the endocardium and spreads through and outwards to the epicardium. It also is propagated at a different velocity from the depolarization wave, and therefore has a different amplitude and length of duration than the QRS wave. Since the repolarization wave moves in the opposite direction from the depolarization wave, its polarity is the same as the QRS complex. The T wave has one particular use during anaesthesia for vascular surgery. Tall T waves —the size of the QRS complex or taller—indicate hyperkalaemia (Lee, 1980). During emergency rapid transfusions of large volumes of blood which is not quite fresh, the level of ionized potassium can rise. (Even under ideal storage conditions the potassium in the red cells of stored blood gradually leaches out into the supernatant serum. Although rewarming the blood whilst it is being transfused into the patient helps reduce the serum potassium level of the transfused blood, it does not complete the process.) The T wave will therefore indicate whether this rise is excessive.

The principal uses for the ECG during anaesthesia for patients undergoing vascular surgery are four:

1. To use as a simple heart rate meter.
2. To determine whether there are any conduction defects caused by the anaesthetic agent—this is less of a problem now that the use of inhalational vapours which are toxic to the myocardium is virtually a thing of the past.
3. For the detection of, and to enable an estimate to be made of the frequency of, ventricular ectopic beats.
4. To provide an opportunity to determine if there is more than one type of ectopic beat.

If the ectopic waves are dissimilar, this indicates that there is more than one abnormal focus and this is much more significant clinically (and more dangerous) than a single aberrant focus that occasionally discharges. The higher the frequency of ventricular ectopic beats, or the greater the number of ectopic foci, the nearer is the onset of ventricular fibrillation.

During the depolarization phase the heart muscle fibre is absolutely refractory to any extraneous electrical impulse including a DC defib-rillation shock. During repolarization, the heart passes through a phase where it is relatively refractory, although if the impulse is big enough—say the equivalent of the work done in passing 100 A (amps) through a 1 ohm resistor for 1 minute or 100 J (joules)—will depolar-ize the heart. This period lasts from 80–120 ms after the QRS com-plex. The heart then becomes very sensitive and an externally applied stimulus of only 10 J (Lown et al., 1973) will be enough to depolarize the heart. It is at this phase that microvolt electrocution can take place. This is the phenomenon where, by chance, a very small voltage current passes through the heart without having an opportunity of dispersing its area of contact with a larger internal body surface. If the electrical current is conducted within a non-conductive plastic tube up to the entrance of the heart—such as by a central venous catheter containing a salt solution—and it strikes the endocardium during the very sensitive phase of the cardiac cycle then, remote though the probability is, this is the time when microvolt electrocution can occur. The source of the current is the reservoir of salt solution and its associated tubing acting as an aerial to collect a powerful radio frequency such as could be emitted from a nearby diathermy machine. If the tip of the catheter is remote from the heart, the current is dispersed over a wider portion of the body before it passes through the heart and the risk of microvolt electrocution is lessened. Better still, any catheter near the heart should contain a non-conduct-ing fluid, or a fluid with a high internal resistance such as a dextrose solution.

Cardiac resuscitation

It is an unfortunate fact of life that any anaesthetist dealing with a reasonably large number of patients with vascular disease will very likely have to resuscitate patients because of the development of either ventricular tachycardia or ventricular fibrillation. These patients are at very high risk as many of them have abnormal coronary arterial trees. The minor malaises of general anaesthesia—a transient hypoxia, a brief period of hypotension—are withstood very badly in these patients. Further, these patients are at risk of developing a coronary occlusion at any time, including during anaesthesia and surgery, which can end up as ventricular fibrillation.

The objective of defibrillation is to apply a large electrical impulse across the heart such that every heart muscle fibre is depolarized simultaneously. Since the repolarization phase lasts for approxi-mately the same time for all heart muscle fibres when the repolari-zation process is complete, all the fibres are then in an optimum condition to receive and react to a normal stimulus from the sinoatrial node to produce a co-ordinated muscle contraction and thereby re-establish normal rhythm. If some of the fibres are in the absolutely refractory phase when the defibrillation impulse is applied, the mass simultaneous depolarization of all the heart muscle fibres will not occur.

In ventricular tachycardia the heart muscle is contracting in a co-ordinated manner but just going too fast. The defibrillation impulse is best applied about 100 ms after the onset of an R wave. A period of asystole lasting a few seconds will then occur. This will allow some metabolic recovery from the local acidosis that has built up within the heart muscle from the excessive work of ventricular tachycardia as well as allowing the fibres to regain more potassium ions which have leached out during the ventricular tachycardia. Both of these factors will help to promote a more stable resting membrane potential and therefore a more normal rhythm.

In ventricular fibrillation the fibres are not contracting in a co-ordinated manner. If the ventricular fibrillation is a fine one, characterized by low-voltage high-frequency waves as seen on the oscilloscope, the degree of inco-ordination is very severe. Any defibrillation stimulus applied is likely to find a number of fibres that are absolutely refractory and therefore resistant to the defibrillation shock. The probability of reversing the fibrillation process is therefore very small. On the other hand, coarse ventricular fibrillation is characterized by larger voltage waves of a lower frequency. This indicates that there are significant masses of muscle fibres acting together, albeit out of phase with other masses. The probability of the defibrillation shock finding significant numbers of fibres absolutely refractory is then very much less and so the likelihood of a successful outcome to the resuscitation is very much higher. The first aim of the resuscitation is therefore to convert any fine ventricular fibrillation into a coarse one and this is best achieved by maximum coronary arterial oxygenation with cardiac massage, plus the liberal supply of alkali salts, calcium ions and beta-stimulating drugs.

After defibrillation, the heart is asystolic for a few seconds. Rather than staring at the oscilloscope waiting for the appearance of some form of cardiac rhythm, cardiac massage should be maintained for a few beats in order to maximize the supply of oxygen to the quiescent heart. This further improves the metabolic chemistry, thereby improving the chances of the restoration of normal rhythm when the heart has recovered from the mass depolarization.

CARDIAC OUTPUT AND OXYGEN FLUX

The prime purpose of the cardiac output is to ensure that there is an adequate despatch of oxygenated blood to the rest of the body. The normal cardiac output is 5 l/min. Blood normally has a haemoglobin concentration of 150 g/l, and each gram is capable of combining with approximately 1·35 ml of oxygen (the amount will vary very slightly depending upon such factors as the pH, P_{CO_2}, temperature, quality of the haemoglobin, etc.). When this combination between oxygen and haemoglobin has been completed, the haemoglobin is fully saturated with oxygen. When the patient is breathing air, the arterial blood is 96–97% saturated with oxygen, slightly less in older patients or in patients with a high left atrial pressure. Putting all these together, the amount of oxygen that is carried through the aortic valve can be calculated according to the following equation:

$$\begin{aligned}
\text{Oxygen flux} \quad &= \text{Cardiac output} \quad \times \text{\% saturation} \quad \times 1·35 \times \text{Hb g/l} \\
&= 5000 \qquad\qquad\quad \times 96/100 \qquad\quad \times 1·35 \times 150/1000 \\
&= 1000 \text{ ml/min approximately}
\end{aligned}$$

Mixed venous blood, after allowance is made for the Bohr effect of pH and carbon dioxide, is 75% saturated. Since at equilibrium the venous return is the same as the cardiac output, this means that the body is consuming 250 ml of oxygen per minute. During anaesthesia the metabolic rate falls. At the Minimum Alveolar Concentration of an anaesthetic gas or vapour which will suppress a somatic reflex response to a surgical stimulus, or MAC1, the metabolic rate falls by about 10% at normothermia. The mixed venous blood is still 75% saturated (again after applying the appropriate correction factors), thus the oxygen flux has also fallen by 10% and this is entirely due to a fall in cardiac output of 10%. At deeper levels of anaesthesia, the fall in flux may be greater than the fall in metabolic rate depending upon the degree of myocardial depression produced by the different anaesthetic agents. At MAC1 all modern inhalational anaesthetic agents depress the cardiac output more or less equally (Hickey and Eger, 1981), but at higher concentrations of anaesthetic the myocardial depression deepens with some anaesthetic agents depressing the heart more than others.

Since the oxygen flux is the product of three factors multiplied together, if all three fall together the effects will be compounded. Thus a reduction of 10% in cardiac output and in oxygen saturation and in haemoglobin concentration will reduce the oxygen flux to about 72% of normal. This is lower than the oxygen content of the normal venous return. A lower haemoglobin concentration of 12 g% or 120 g/l combined with a 10% fall in cardiac output will produce an oxygen flux of 70% of normal—yet this particular combination is not uncommon in the elderly arteriosclerotic patient. Such patients are also frequently mildly hypoxaemic due to the hypoxaemia of age (Marshall and Wyche, 1972). Putting this all together, these patients have a marked reduction in their reserves of oxygen supply.

The average extraction rate of oxygen for the body as a whole is 25% of the normal supply. Some tissues, notably the heart have a higher extraction rate; the heart has a 66% extraction rate (Little, 1981c) whilst the brain has a 33% extraction rate, although this varies sharply and non-linearly with increasing depth of anaesthesia (Stullken et al., 1977). Applying the same calculations of oxygen flux to the heart, a 10% reduction in coronary artery flow combined with a mild anaemia to 12 g% halves the reserve of oxygen that is available to the heart as a whole. This reserve is the excess of supply over demand. But the 66% extraction rate is the average for the whole heart, and some parts of the heart work harder than others, notably the left ventricle where the extraction rate is over 75%. Any mild degree of hypoxaemia will compound the issue to the point of no oxygen reserve at all. The coronary vessels are well endowed with vasodilator nerve fibres (Little, 1981b) and they respond to hypoxaemia by inducing vasodilatation of the coronary artery circulation to increase the coronary blood flow and this will augment the oxygen flux. However, the patient with severe degenerative or occlusive coronary artery disease may be at a significant disadvantage—he may already be maximally vasodilated and so may not be able to compensate for any change in oxygen sypply. As the coronary vessels become more and more pressure dependent, they are unable to develop a pattern of low pressure hyperaemia of a vasodilated bed and thus they become more and more vulnerable to any change in oxygen supply.

The normal response to chronic anaemia is to increase the cardiac output. The mechanism by which this is sensed is unknown, although involvement of oxygen tension sensors on the right side of the heart has been considered. The effect of this response is an increase in the work of the heart. This increase is not linear with the reduction in haemoglobin content; it is offset slightly by the reduced viscosity of anaemic blood. Nevertheless, the increase in work done does mean an increase in oxygen demand.

Apart from responding to changes in pH, $Paco_2$ and Po_2 the cardiac output also changes with changes in the depth of anaesthesia. At MAC1 there is a 10% reduction in cardiac output, deeper levels of MAC by inhalational agents further depress the cardiac output but the extent will then depend upon the particular inhalational anaesthetic agents. Thiopentone depresses the cardiac output, whilst methohexitone, in high doses, increases the cardiac output by lowering the peripheral resistance very substantially (Wise et al., 1969). Hypothermia reduces the cardiac output 10% per °C after due allowance has been made for any changes in pH or Rosenthal effect (Rosenthal, 1948) and $Paco_2$ or Severinghaus effect with temperature (Severinghaus, 1966). Tubocurarine depresses the cardiac output somewhat, whilst pancuronium increases it, although the magnitude of these effects are very slight. A single dose of succinylcholine has no effect on cardiac output, but repetitive doses gradually reduce it and may transiently abolish it (Bullough, 1959; Tomlin and Duck, 1975). Atropine increases the cardiac output, mainly through removing any parasympathetic inhibition, whilst neostigmine has the reverse effect depending upon the degree of anti-muscarinic protection previously given. The cardiac output could fall to zero if a large dose of neostigmine is given intravenously to an unprotected heart.

FACTORS AFFECTING THE DISTRIBUTION OF THE CARDIAC OUTPUT

The cardiac output is distributed to the different tissues, each of which is capable of adjusting its supply according to need. 5% goes to the heart (Wade and Bishop, 1962), 12·5–15% goes to the brain, 10% goes directly to the liver via the hepatic artery (and a highly variable 24% will go indirectly to the liver via the bowel and portal system, the variation being due to whether there is need for an increase in blood supply to pick up food and take it to the liver for reprocessing). One-fifth goes to the kidneys although here too this is in excess of the kidneys' metabolic needs, the excess being for filtration purposes. It is the gut and renal blood flow that constitutes much of the reserve that is called upon in the event of a sudden severe blood loss. There is, in addition, 10% of the body's blood volume in the lungs and pulmonary vascular bed at any instant of time (Keele et al., 1982a) which contributes to the body's reserve of blood.

Coronary flow

Although normally only 5% of the cardiac output goes to the heart, when the heart is working harder this proportion is increased. The coronary vessels have a capacity of increasing their flow up to five-fold (Berne and Rubrio, 1979). In the arteriopathic patient not only is there hypertension and the need to increase contractility because the after-load impedance has increased and the diastolic pump is less effective so that the heart is working harder, but the capacity to expand even further the coronary inflow may be limited, i.e. the reserve may be only as high as threefold or as low as nil.

Cerebral flow

At 750 ml/min the brain receives some 15% of the cardiac output (Kety and Schmidt, 1948). Despite this, the oxygen extraction rate is 33%. This extraction rate is virtually constant, whether awake and thinking furiously or relaxing with eyes closed (Fieschi and Lenzi, 1983), i.e. the overwhelming bulk of the cerebral oxygen supply is for housekeeping purposes to keep the neurones alive. The most highly perfused of the brain substance is the reticular formation of the brain stem (Little, 1981b). The most vulnerable portions of the brain to generalized hypoxia (as after a cardiac arrest in a previously healthy brain with a normal vascular bed) are the dorsomedial portions of the midbrain, the occipital cortex and the basal ganglia, in that order (Stephenson, 1974). The pons and medulla are the most resistant portions of the brain to hypoxia—they can survive after a cardiac arrest when all the remaining brain cells have died, but this survival does depend upon the pons and medulla being reasonably well oxygenated before the episode of cerebral circulatory standstill. Pre-existing zones of relative ischaemia, as in cerebro-atherosclerosis, can change dramatically the pattern of neurone survival after an episode of cerebral circulatory standstill.

There appear to be no functional vasodilator or vasoconstrictor nerve fibres to the vessels in the distribution of the internal carotid or basilar arteries. Although the cerebral vasculature is richly innervated by branches of the superior cervical ganglion, yet the resting sympathetic tone is minimal. The role of the sympathetic nerves in the regulation of cerebral blood flow is unclear (Heistad and Kontos, 1983). There are some vasodilator fibres in the distribution of the external carotoid artery and these follow the anastomoses between the external and internal carotid trees at the junction of the dura and cerebral cortex and may penetrate for up to 1 cm into the cerebral cortex. It follows, therefore, that cerebral blood flow is dependent entirely on two factors: the applied pressure and the cerebral vascular resistance. Certain anaesthetics, notably the volatile agents, increase cerebral blood flow by reducing the vascular resistance notwithstanding the reduction in blood pressure that they can cause. Halothane is the worst offender in this respect (McDowall, 1965). This is of clinical significance during anaesthesia for cerebral angiography when the clinician is trying to ascertain if there is a cerebral aneurysm.

The principal factors affecting cerebral blood flow are the Pa_{CO_2} and the Pa_{O_2}, but only if the haemoglobin concentration is normal. Brown and his co-workers (Brown et al., 1985) have found that when evaluating patients with a wide range of haemoglobin concentrations the key factor in determining the cerebral blood flow was the oxygen content, not oxygen tension, of the arterial blood. In severe anaemia the cerebral blood flow was high despite a high oxygen tension, and conversely in polycythaemic patients the cerebral blood flow was lower than expected for any given oxygen tension. Varying the viscosity made little difference. It appeared that the system was operating to maintain a constant supply of oxygen to the brain, presumably if this fell then locally produced metabolites induced vasodilatation. Such a system would, of course, obviate the need for special oxygen tension sensors in the cerebral circulation. In the patient with severe cerebral-atherosclerosis this system would appear to fail in that the cerebral blood flow in these patients is much more pressure dependent and viscosity dependent (McHenry et al., 1974). Given a normal haemoglobin, a high Pa_{CO_2} or a low Pa_{O_2} will cause very marked cerebral vasodilatation whereas the converse, a low Pa_{CO_2} or high Pa_{O_2}, will cause vasoconstriction. Providing the exposure is not unduly prolonged, at normal atmospheric pressure the high Pa_{O_2} effects are of little consequence except in the newborn, when the problems of retrolental fibroplasia occur. Under hyperbaric conditions a high Pa_{O_2} will provoke sufficient cerebral vasoconstriction as to cause serious disorientation (Lamberton, 1980). The vasoconstrictive effects of a low Pa_{CO_2} can be much more harmful. This is particularly true if there is an area of cerebro-atherosclerosis and there has been chronic carbon dioxide retention. Although a high Pa_{CO_2} provokes vasodilatation, after a period of time there is some adaptation and the cerebral blood flow reverts to normal. Enthusiastic artificial ventilation to lower the Pa_{CO_2} to more conventional limits will then provoke sufficient cerebral ischaemia as to cause clinically significant neuronal dysfunction (Froman, 1968) if not depopulation. This situation is enhanced if there is cerebro-atherosclerosis. Pumping blood past a partial occlusion will consume energy and distal to the occlusion the pressure will be lower. If the run-off is then impaired by an increase in resistance, consequent upon small vessel constriction, flow will be reduced. This is further favoured by the elastic recoil of these small vessels. The smaller the diameter, the higher is the critical opening pressure necessary to establish flow (Burton, 1962) so that stagnation and thrombus formation are more likely. This is relevant to the anaesthetic management of patients undergoing vascular surgery—especially where there is evidence of cerebro-atherosclerosis, as in patients undergoing carotid endarterectomy. Excessive artificial ventilation in these patients prejudices neuronal function (as seen in the EEG) and eventually neuronal survival.

Renal flow

In the patient with vascular disease, the results of drastic changes in renal blood flow can be critical, yet the renal flow is an important reserve in conserving blood flow to the essential organs (the heart, liver and brain) in the event of sudden blood loss. Many patients with vascular disease have minor degrees of renal failure. This is in part due to the general effects of old age (Kalchthaler, 1978) but also in part as one of the consequences of hypertension. Atheromatous plaques causing partial obstruction to the renal blood flow mean that renal vasoconstriction, arising from an attempt to compensate for severe blood loss, will lead to stasis. Total renal infarction is a very real risk. With lesser degrees of vascular occlusion, it may not be possible to maintain the orderly redistribution of the reduced blood flow through the different parts of the kidneys, e.g. via the arcuate arteries and other vessels that are necessary for the preservation of the renal tubules. Some renal tubules will not receive any oxygen and will die. Renal tubular necrosis is proportionately much more common in patients undergoing vascular surgery who have a serious fall in cardiac output. In some centres it is the commonest indication for emergency haemodialysis. Minor degrees of renal damage are much more common and elevations of the serum creatinine level are almost an invariable consequence of a hypotensive episode during anaesthesia and surgery in vascular patients.

FLOW, PRESSURE AND RESISTANCE

In the normal subject blood leaves the heart at a mean velocity of 40 cm/s or $1\frac{1}{2}$ ft/s or 1 mile/h, rising to a peak of 120 cm/s (Ganong 1983b). The peak flow, apart from a very brief overshoot as the aortic valve opens, is approximately 200 ml/s and this is sustained as a square wave for about 0·2 s and gradually subsides to a dichrotic notch to deliver a stroke volume of 70 ml over a period of 0·4–0·5 s. Then, flow through the aortic valve ceases until the next systole. This is not true for other areas of the circulation. After the dichrotic notch, the flow varies with the site of sensing. At the root of the aorta reverse flow is seen as the diastolic pump discharges blood into the coronary vessels, whilst at the level of the diaphragm forward flow is seen during the diastolic period due to the diastolic recoil of the elastic upper aorta (*Fig.* 1.2).

The average velocity of blood in the descending aorta is 20–25 cm/s, due to the spreading effect of the diastolic pump maintaining flow during diastole and saving a considerable amount of energy.

The velocity of flow in any stream is, among other things, a function of the diameter of its containing vessel or tube, the narrower the diameter for the same applied flow and loading pressure the higher is the velocity. Hence the velocity in an injector system increases in the central narrowed stem. The common iliac vessels are narrower than the aorta and, as a consequence, the velocity of flow increases to double, 50 cm/s. This is close to the Reynolds number (Uvarov et al., 1973) at which turbulence develops. Any small partial occlusion, or increase in pressure gradient, will increase the velocity further to the point where turbulence occurs. This, in turn, will lead to mechanical distension and stretching of the vessel which will tend to quench the

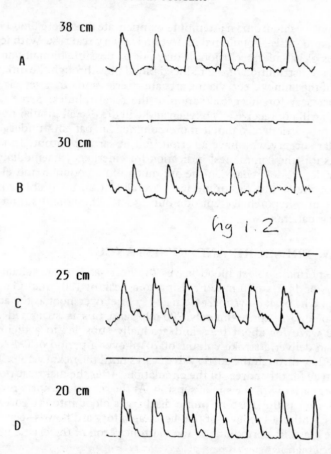

Fig. 1.2. **Flow velocity profiles at different levels in the aorta. Doppler recording in man of aortic blood velocity at different distances from the incisor teeth. Trace A is a recording from just above the diaphragm. Trace B was taken from mid-thorax level. The multiphasic tracing C is at the level of the aortic arch and is typical of the pattern resulting from turbulent flow. In patients with severe arterial disease this pattern of turbulence persists from the aortic arch to the crus of the diaphragm. Tracing D shows the velocity wave in the common carotid.**

(Reproduced with acknowledgements from Tomlin P. J. and Duck F. A. (1975) Transoesophageal aortovelography in man. *Can. Anaesth. Soc. J.* **22**: 561.)

turbulence, but the turbulence will further increase the atheromatous deposition and this will lead to further loss of elasticity and further narrowing.

Blood flow in the descending aorta is neither turbulent nor laminar. Analysis of the back-reflected, Doppler-shifted ultrasonic signals from a transoesophageal probe (Duck et al., 1974) has shown that there is an extremely narrow range of velocities at any instant of the cardiac cycle (*Fig.* 1.3); over 95% of the flow is travelling at the same speed whilst the bow wave of systole is rectangular, i.e. blood flows as a bolus and any intravenous drug, or dye used for the dye dilution method of estimating cardiac output, is also moving as a bolus whilst in the arterial system. This change in profile from the expected laminar pattern is due to the distensibility of the elastic walls of the aorta.

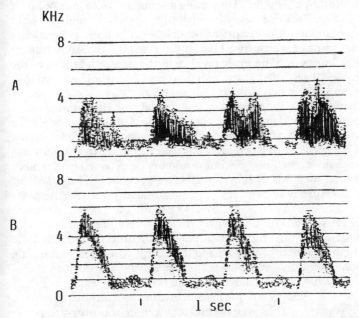

Fig. 1.3. **Frequency spectrum of blood velocity in bolus and turbulent flow in man. Trace B is from a normal subject. In early systole all the blood travels at the same speed, i.e. at any instant in time there is no scatter of velocities. Later in systole there is some scatter of velocities but the scatter is low and the grey scale of frequency intensity shows that 90 + % of the blood if at the same speed, i.e. there is negligible lamination, the blood is flowing as a bolus at varying speeds during systole.**

In contrast trace A is turbulent flow with a complete range of velocities at all times during systole. The velocities are of random intensity. Flow is totally turbulent.

(Reproduced with acknowledgements from Duck F. A., Hodson C. J. and Tomlin P. J. (1974) An oesophageal probe for aortic flow velocity monitoring. *Ultrasound Med. Biol.* **3**: 233. Pergamon Press.)

Pressure waves travel faster than flow waves. A pressure wave travelling through a fluid contained in a rigid container will travel at the speed of sound in that fluid. As the container becomes more elastic so the velocity of a pressure wave is reduced. The 95% frequency response (Gersh et al., 1971) is lengthened and the result is some degradation and dampening of the original pressure signal. Simultaneous pressure signals recorded from the root of the aorta and the periphery show this degradation very well; the main differences seen at the periphery are a slower rise of the pressure wave at the beginning of systole and a rounding of the main wave to nearer a sinusoid pattern with a dichrotic notch. The average velocity of the pressure wave in the subject with normal arteries is a little over 600 cm/s. In contrast in the atherosclerotic patient the dampening is much less to the point of non-existence. Pressure waves travel at high speeds through the rigid arteries bouncing off every major branch, each bounce generating a reflection, some of which travel back up the arterial tree so that there may be 3, 4 or even 5 dichrotic notches in the descending part of the pressure signal recorded at the radial artery. The whole arterial system is ringing like a bell with every heart beat.

Another effect of the rigidity of the arterial tree is the initial overshoot in pressure and flow that occurs at the root of the aorta when the aortic valve opens can be transmitted to the periphery and sensed there. This spike or high pressure may last no more than 0·05 s and can be seen on an oscilloscope (but would not be detected by the more conventional methods of measuring blood pressure). This transient spike of pressure is so brief that the mean blood pressure (the pressure averaged over a period of time) is virtually unchanged. Accurate peak digital voltmeters will display this as a very high pressure and this can be of concern to the uninitiated. The duration of this little flick of high pressure is too short and the energy it contains is too little to have any disruptive effect—whether on an arterial suture or a cerebral vessel. A high mean arterial pressure is much more sinister in this respect and if the spike is prolonged in time it will raise the mean arterial pressure. In the assessment of whether the pressure is too high, the clinician must have some idea of the shape and the duration of the pressure wave and this can only be obtained by a visual display of the analogue signal on an oscilloscope screen.

The systolic blood pressure is the highest lateral hydrostatic pressure exerted against the walls of the artery during the cardiac cycle. The diastolic pressure is the lowest pressure within the arteries during the cardiac cycle. The mean arterial pressure is the average pressure exerted against the walls of the artery over a period of time. The pulse pressure is the difference between the systolic and diastolic pressure.

The aortic impedance is the instantaneous resistance against the forward flow of blood in the aorta. It is variable during the cardiac cycle, reaching a maximum at peak systolic flow. Conventionally, the aortic impedance is the ratio of oscillatory pressure and oscillatory flow (O'Rourke, 1982b). To calculate it one must subtract the steady work from the total work. The steady work is the mean arterial pressure multiplied by the stroke volume—this is the work that would be required to maintain constant flow through the peripheral resistance. The total work is the sum of the pressure flow work and the kinetic work. The pressure flow work is the integral or sum of the product of instantaneous flow and pressure, whilst the kinetic work is the integral of the product of the square of the instantaneous velocity and stroke volume, that is,

Pulsatile work = Total work − steady work
Total work = Pressure flow work + kinetic work
Pressure flow work = Sum of instantaneous pressure × flow
Kinetic work = Stroke volume × sum of square of
instantaneous velocity
(or mass × velocity squared approximately)
Steady work = Mean pressure × stroke volume

so that

Pulsatile work = Pressure flow work + kinetic work − steady
work
$$= \int (P \times V) + SV \times \int (Vel)^2 - (Mean\ P \times SV)$$
where   V = Instantaneous flow
Vel = Instantaneous velocity
SV = Stroke Volume
P = Instantaneous pressure

The ratio of pulsatile work to total work is the proportion of work spent on pulsatile losses (O'Rourke, 1967). It will be appreciated that in the patient with arterial disease the mean arterial pressure will have risen, but not by the same proportion as the systolic pressure —as diastolic pressure only rises slightly (10–20% compared with 40–60% for the systolic pressure). Stroke volume is unchanged. Therefore the steady work has increased only a little. Because of the reduction if not loss of the diastolic pump effect, the velocity has increased and therefore the kinetic work has increased considerably as it increases with the square of the velocity. Meanwhile, the instantaneous pressure also has increased, from the peak of the raised systolic pressure, so that the pressure flow work has increased substantially. The ratio of pulsatile work to total work increases—that is, pulsatile losses as a fraction of the total work increase: there is a marked increase in aortic impedance in the patient with degenerative vascular disease.

The peripheral resistance is the average resistance to the average flow of blood through the circulation and is the difference between the mean arterial pressure and the mean venous pressure divided by the cardiac output. It is measured in units of force per unit flow per unit cross-sectional area (Green, 1944) and since force is dynes (or Newtons) and flow is volume per second, it is expressed as dyne $.\,s\,.\,cm^{-5}$. The normal peripheral resistance is between 1000 and 1500 resistance units (dynes per square cm per unit of flow) but in patients with arterial disease it is usually significantly elevated. In S. I. units the most convenient description of the normal values is $100-150\,kPa\,.\,l^{-1}\,.\,s^{-1}$.

Blood pressure is the product of the cardiac output and peripheral resistance. If one falls and the other rises there will be little change in blood pressure, although the heart rate will have changed. The clinical significance of a change in cardiac output compared with a change in peripheral resistance is very different. A fall in cardiac output is rarely to the patient's advantage, whereas given an unchanged blood pressure a fall in peripheral resistance means that there is an increase in flow—that is, there has been an increase in the supply of oxygen etc. to the tissues.

The blood pressure is controlled by a number of subsystems. In the arch of the aorta, at the origins of the major vessels and the carotid sinus are stretch receptors (Heymans and Neil, 1958) which respond to pulsatile distension to increase the sympathetic discharge to the heart in the event of hypotension, and reduce the sympathetic discharge in the event of hypertension. In man, no one part is particularly dominant, e.g. reducing the inflow to the carotid sinus during carotid endarterectomy has little effect, *per se*, on the activity of the heart. It is the sum of the output of all these sensors, acting through the vasomotor centre, which is the major determinant of blood pressure control in the normal subject.

The most important effector subsystem is the peripheral arteriole and its sympathetic nerve supply. The peripheral arteriole is sensitive to hypoxia and acidosis. Both lower the effects of the sympathetic discharge on the arteriole and so favour local vasodilatation. Changes in posture also impose a hydrostatic stress on the circulation, with the risk of excessive flow to the dependent parts. The vasomotor centre acting through the arterioles ensures that this does not happen. A spectacular example is the very large size of the arteriole, and its control, in the ankle of the giraffe—an animal whose intracranial mean arterial pressure is the same as that in man (Warren, 1974). But the intracranial arteriole is positioned some 15–18 ft above the ankle, so that the arteriole in the ankle is exposed to a pressure of 450–550 mmHg (90 mmHg plus 15 ft of water or its equivalent, half an atmosphere of pressure). Hence the arteriole in the ankle of the giraffe has to be very substantial to withstand this pressure and not allow an excessive blood flow to the foot when the animal is erect, and yet be capable of maintaining the flow when the hydrostatic pressure is lessened as when the animal lowers its thorax to drink.

In normal man, three-quarters of the changes in blood pressure occurring between when the blood leaves the heart and when it returns to the heart occur at the arterioles (Little, 1981c). The diameter of the arterioles is therefore of crucial importance in sustaining the peripheral resistance. This diameter is controlled by smooth muscle fibres arranged circularly around the vessel and innervated by the sympathetic nerve fibres. Sympathetic nervous system activity raises the tonus of the muscle, thereby increasing its tension and so narrowing the diameter, unless opposed by the intraluminal pressure. Some nerve fibres can lower the tonus of the muscle thus enabling the arteriole to distend in response to an increase in intraluminal pressure. As the tension within the circular muscle rises, the intraluminal pressure required to overcome this rises very considerably. If the tension is high enough, the vessel shuts down tight to produce zero flow. The minimum pressure required to re-establish flow is the critical opening pressure (Burton, 1962). This minimum opening pressure is dictated in part by the elastic fibres in the wall of the arterioles—which behave like elastic tissue anywhere, that is, it requires a relatively large force to induce some stretching, but thereafter further stretching requires less effort—and in part by the tonus of the arteriolar muscle. Reducing the level of sympathetic drive reduces the tonus at the arteriole and with it the critical opening pressure.

In the patient with severe vascular disease, the circulatory system is much more pressure sensitive, with the main emphasis of sustaining blood pressure relying on the cardiac output (and with this the venous return). With many sclerosed or partially occluded vessels, the sympathetic vasoconstrictor tone is reduced to a minimum, whilst sympathetic vasodilator fibres have opened up many collateral vessels in an often vain attempt to respond to a demand for a restoration of a flow of oxygenated blood to the ischaemic tissues. The ability to lower the peripheral resistance by further vasodilatation is therefore limited. This is why there is often only a marginal improvement in flow and little change in blood pressure during lumbar sympathectomy, even though the small increment in flow may be enough to ensure viability of a limb.

Another effect also comes into play. Arterioles subject to sustained hypertension undergo slow structural changes, muscle hypertrophy, hyalinization, medial necrosis and degeneration and replacement by fibrous tissue. All this leads to a protection of the distal capillary bed from being exposed to high pressures (Walter and Israel, 1979) and without a constant energy demand and autonomic system supervision of the arteriolar muscle. This is most clearly seen in the pulmonary circulation when there is chronic pulmonary hypertension as a result of mitral stenosis (where it is necessary to protect the alveolae from pulmonary oedema) but it happens throughout the body. Those arterioles arising from arteries which do not have significant patches of occlusive atheroma are particularly exposed to the hypertension. As a result of the increasing rigidity of these arterioles consequent upon these structural changes, their ability to vasoconstrict or dilate is impaired. The flexibility in altering the size of the vascular bed to accommodate changes in circulating blood volume becomes progressively less. This throws further reliance on the cardiac output and myocardial contractility to maintain the blood pressure. Since the cardiac output cannot exceed the venous return, apart from the limited reserve in the pulmonary circulation, the arterial blood pressure in the patient with vascular disease then becomes a sensitive indicator of the circulating blood volume.

PERIPHERAL FLOW

Part of the frictional resistance to the forward flow of blood is the viscosity of the blood itself. Blood is not a simple Newtonian fluid but a suspension of cells in plasma. In the larger vessels, this effect is of little consequence. In the smaller vessels, those of a diameter of approximately $\times 50$ the diameter of a red cell or less, there develops axial streaming of the red cells, with only pure plasma in contact with the vessel wall. Viscosity increases with haematocrit (Pirofsky, 1953). This process of plasma skimming means that the viscous drag is then much less and is almost entirely at the plasma–vessel wall boundary. The viscosity of blood in the capillaries is thus close to that of plasma (Keele et al., 1982b). Changing the characteristics of the plasma by diluting it with a colloid, e.g. the dextrans, can marginally reduce this viscosity and therefore improve flow through the small vessels. Diluting the plasma with a simple salt solution confers no useful benefit as this is comparatively rapidly excreted by the kidneys.

Flow through the arteriole is dependent upon the peripheral run-off through the capillaries and postcapillary vessels. The postcapillary vessels are the venous resistance vessels and they also are well endowed with sympathetic nerves. If these venous resistance vessels have too high a resistance, there will be tissue engorgement and tissue oedema.

Between the arteriole and venuole is the network of capillaries, some of which pass straight to the venuole, others wind their way back tortuously (Zweifach, 1939; Ham, 1969a) around the tissues before joining the venuole. Flow can be sluggish, as the blood meanders through many capillaries giving a lot of time for oxygen exchange, or flow can be fast, as it darts through the precapillary shunts. In the case of the skin, the meandering also provides time for offloading excessive heat. If there is a need to conserve heat, the precapillary shunt vessels open wide, minimizing capillary skin perfusion. Entry to these shunt vessels is heavily influenced by the sympathetic system. Under anaesthesia, this shunt control is much reduced; there is a marked increase in capillary flow, although the extent of the cutaneous vasodilatation varies with the different inhalational agents (Hickey and Eger, 1981). As a result, heat control is lost and there is significant redistribution of the body heat, with loss of heat from the central core and a gain of heat in the subcutaneous tissues.

The capillaries are not closed tubes of flat pavement cells. There are spiral clefts between the cells (Ham, 1969b) which allow for the escape of fluid and ions but the clefts are not normally big enough to allow protein to pass through. If the capillaries have become severely hypoxaemic or there has been trauma, either chemical or physical, the pavement cells swell. This increases the size of the intercellular clefts, as the turgid pavement cells separate. This, in turn, leads to a protein-containing oedema. Excessive metabolism, as after severe exercise, can have much the same effect (Starling, 1898). The clefts between the endothelial cells of the liver are large, so that hepatic extracellular fluid has a 2% protein content, whereas resting muscle has no protein in its extracellular fluid although the extracellular fluid from a heavily exercising muscle may have as much as 1–2% protein content.

Another factor that helps maintain the microcirculation and the peripheral flow is the electrostatic charge on the red cells, and platelets. Normal red cells have a small excess of 10 µV negative charge within the cells. Electrostatic repulsion helps to keep the red cells separate. The pavement endothelium also has a repulsive charge aimed at keeping the particles to within the plasma stream. Following trauma, the charge falls—the mechanisms by which this is achieved are unknown. The red cells tend to adhere to each other more readily, whilst fresh platelets also have a greater adhesiveness. Red cell aggregation then may occur, forming a sticky sludge which significantly diminishes the efficiency of flow in the microcirculation (MacLean, 1981; Prentice, 1981). The aggregates are carried around the blood stream. On striking a mechanical obstruction the red cells may not disaggregate, but may form an obstructive plug to an arteriole. Some may be swept through the postarteriolar shunt to end in the lungs (where they make a contribution to the shock lung syndrome), but the majority remain in the peripheral tissues. Here, they normally do little harm, as minor order collateral vessels maintain peripheral oxygenation until the aggregates are scavenged away. But white cells and platelets can, in addition to red cells, pile up on the aggregates to form microthrombi. It is only if this is on an extensive scale that the result is diffuse intravascular coagulation. This serious coagulopathy is thus only one end of a spectrum that ranges from a minor to a major disorder.

THE VENOUS RETURN

The venuoles are formed by capillaries joining together. As they approach 0·5 mm in diameter a thin circular muscle coat forms around them (Ham, 1969b). This is the postcapillary sphincter. The pressure within the vessel is low—little more than the plasma protein osmotic pressure—so the tone of the muscle is low. A small increase in the muscle tone of this sphincter can therefore have a marked effect on the flow within the venuole and cause local oedema.

The circular coat continues all the length of the vein, whilst the long veins, e.g. of the leg, acquire a longitudinal muscle layer (Ham, 1969c). The muscles of the veins are heavily innervated by sympathetic nerves—there are no parasympathetic fibres to the veins. The function of the sympathetic nerves is to maintain the venous muscle tone. Venous vasodilatation occurs as a result of a lowering of the venous tone, which can be local or general.

At any instant of time, approximately 80% of the circulating blood volume is within the veins (Little, 1981d). Because the system is a low pressure system relative to the volume contained, any small reduction in venous vasomotor tone has a marked effect on the capacity of the veins to hold more blood without changing the intraluminal pressure. This has led to the confusion over whether there are separate capacitance vessels and resistance vessels within the venous system (Rothe, 1983). In fact there is a continuous gradation of effect due to the degree of sympathetic activity, but the essence of the venous system is that it is a very compliant one.

Flow and pressure within the veins are subject to a number of factors. These are the *vis a frontae* (which is the hydrostatic pressure of the column of blood opposing the centripetal movement of the flow of blood), the *vis lateralis* (which is the lateral pressure exerted on the blood flow, in part due to the muscle of the vein wall and in part due to the compressive action of the muscles of the limbs and trunk) and the *vis a tergo* (the residual of the pressure generated by the heart and mainly, but not completely, dissipated during the passage of the blood through the arterioles and capillaries). Centripetal movement of the blood is aided by the presence of valves, even by the incomplete valves that are within the large veins.

The *vis a frontae* changes markedly as the blood approaches the chest. The hydrostatic effect of the column of blood is obviously smaller, but within the chest there are also other pressures being generated by the act of breathing. Each spontaneous respiration generates a subatmospheric pressure within the chest. The *vis a frontae* then becomes transiently negative and this enhances the forward movement of the blood. It is for this reason that peripheral venous pressure measurement cannot substitute for central venous pressure measurement.

As the column of blood approaches the thorax it develops three pressure waves per cardiac cycle. These are the a, c and v waves (Mackay, 1967) and they reflect events within the cardiac cycle. The a wave reflects atrial contraction, the c wave reflects the recoil caused by closure of the tricuspid valve, whilst the v wave reflects the distension to the tricuspid valve produced by the peak intraventricular pressure. The shorter the c wave–v wave interval the more quickly this peak of pressure has been achieved and the better the myocardial contractility. From the c wave on until the end of systole, the baseline pressure of the central veins rises as the venous return continues against the closed tricuspid valve.

Central venous pressure

Central venous pressure is the mean pressure in the veins within the chest. In the horizontal position, if the right atrial pressure is not too low, the neck vein pressure equates with the central venous pressure, so that pressure measurement obtained from the external jugular vein can be used as a substitute for central venous pressure measurement. If the right atrial pressure is low, then the subatmospheric pressure of the spontaneously breathing patient will cause a transient but actual collapse of the veins during inspiration, so that the mean pressure within the external jugular vein no longer reflects the true mean central venous pressure, as the subatmospheric component does not get through to make its contribution to the mean pressure. As a consequence the mean pressure obtained from the external jugular vein reads high, relative to the central venous pressure. During controlled respiration without a negative phase this situation does not apply, as there is then no subatmospheric pressure within the chest. Hence, during controlled respiration the central venous pressure measurement can be obtained from the external jugular vein whilst, but only whilst, the patient is in the horizontal position.

The relationship between right atrial pressure and the venous return is a complex one as the venous return is one of the factors affecting right atrial pressure. If the venous return is high, right ventricular end-diastolic pressure rises. This, via the Starling mechanism, increases the right ventricular output. This, in turn, increases the pulmonary blood flow and then left atrial pressure and left ventricular end-diastolic pressure and left ventricular output. In the extreme situation, eventually left ventricular output fails to match input and a series of back pressure effects builds up with pulmonary hyperaemia (perhaps with oedema), and right ventricular strain and a rising right atrial pressure opposing the venous return. This is high output failure.

At a high but not excessive venous return, moderate back pressure effects cause little disturbance to the venous return, e.g. a raised mean intrathoracic pressure, as in artificial ventilation. A high venous return implies a full circulating blood volume and active sympathetic system acting on the venous tone. The stimulus to myocardial contractility is such that there is little fluctuation in stroke volume or systolic pressure with ventilation, although there is some.

When the venous return is below this high optimum flow, the mean right atrial pressure falls. At around zero pressure, an applied intra-thoracic pressure raises the atrial pressure, opposing venous inflow. At the same time, the pulmonary veins are subject to pressure and this aids the venous return to the left atrium, so that left atrial venous return increases whilst right atrial venous return decreases. The left atrial venous return stretches the left ventricle, causing an increase in the force of contraction and ejection. Stroke volume and stroke pressure therefore rise. This cannot be sustained beyond a few heart beats as the pulmonary inflow is falling. There is, therefore, marked oscillation in systolic blood pressure with respiration, the peaks coinciding with the peaks in central venous pressure. Clinically this swinging of arterial pressure with controlled ventilation (in a closed chest) indicates that the venous return is somewhat below optimal and the patient will cope less well with any sudden or large blood loss. Improving the venous return by increasing the circulating blood volume ameliorates this.

Central venous pressure is sometimes taken as an index of adequacy of the venous return and therefore of the circulating blood volume. This is only true if, for other reasons such as chronic heart failure, the right atrial pressure is chronically raised. Such a heart needs a high right atrial pressure to sustain its output and this is achieved by the patient developing a permanent high resting venomotor tone to sustain a normal venous return. Under these conditions, if the venous return is augmented by a short sharp infusion, the central venous pressure will rise sharply. If the heart is working near its limit, the central venous pressure stays elevated for a good few minutes and further transfusion is not going to help the patient and indeed may push the patient to the inefficient part of the ventricular function curve. If, following a short sharp infusion, the central venous pressure rises sharply but then falls back briskly, then the venous return is below the capacity of the heart to pump it onwards (Sykes, 1963). The need to give further transfusion will then depend upon the clinical assessment of stroke volume and stroke pressure. If, in response to a short sharp infusion, there is little to no change in central venous pressure, then the venous return is almost certainly inadequate and the patient needs further transfusion. This situation works well against a background of a chronically raised right atrial pressure.

In the patient whose right ventricle and right atrium are not chronically stressed, but whose venomotor tone is not particularly active, i.e. when the venous system is very compliant the central venous pressure offers a poor and slow guide to the adequacy of the circulating blood volume and the need for transfusion. In the presence of blood loss, the venomotor tone rises to sustain the venous return, so that the central venous pressure changes little and very slowly—needing 10–20 min before a new equilibrium is achieved.

Such a situation arises during the anaesthetic management of patients with vascular disease. The initial induction agent depresses the venomotor tone, particularly at the level of the postcapillary sphincter; venous vasodilatation results. Cardiac output falls, as does the systemic blood pressure. As the drug wears off, there is no particular stress to activate the venous sympathetic system—although, if the patient is lightly anaesthetized, the stimulus of the surgical incision will do this, but in general the venous sympathetic tone is low. Frequently, it is necessary to expand rapidly the circulating blood volume, by a rapid infusion of crystalloid to compensate for the increase in the size of the vascular bed, in order to maintain the venous return and so the cardiac output and blood pressure. Blood loss is also a venous sympathetic system stimulus and so, if blood loss does occur, the venous pressure is sustained initially. It is only when the circulating blood volume is very markedly depleted that the venous pressure falls severely. In the presence of an adequate circulating blood volume, a short sharp infusion will not produce a sustained rise in central venous pressure as the heart is not near its failing limit. It simply responds via the Starling effect. Thus, within the context of the clinical management of reasonably fit patients undergoing vascular surgery, central venous pressure measurement provides too slow a guide to be particularly valuable during the intra-operative period of a vascular operation. It does provide a useful back-up if there is a slow slide to peripheral vasodilatation. If there is any element of fluid retention, mild chronic heart failure or chronic renal failure, then the central venous pressure is more responsive to changes in the circulating blood volume.

SHOCK

The term 'shock' covers a variety of conditions with widely differing aetiologies and therefore needing quite different therapies but tending, especially near the terminal phase, to end in a final common pathway of progressive circulatory failure and death. One very early investigator described it as 'a momentary pause in the act of death'. Because the therapeutic endeavours are so different the term 'shock', unless qualified, is totally meaningless. It has indeed been called a semantic enigma (Rushmer et al., 1962). There are four different types of shock,

1. Neurogenic shock
2. Hypovolaemic shock
3. Cardiogenic shock
4. Septicaemic shock

NEUROGENIC SHOCK

This is a state of failure of vasomotor control, from failure either of the vasomotor centre or its pathways. As a result, there is loss of vaso-constrictor tone at the arterioles leading to arteriolar vasodilatation and hypotension, with a marked fall in peripheral vascular resistance. The heart is healthy and responds to any change in the venous return but the loss of vasoconstrictive drive, including venous vasoconstric-tive drive, is such that the venous return will depend almost entirely on gravity. If vagal tone is still active, there will be bradycardia and some reduced myocardial contractility. The main causes of neuro-genic shock are spinal cord injuries and anything that might cause coning of the brain stem, such as some intracranial haemorrhages, any source of raised intracranial pressure and pneumo-encephalo-graphy. Clinically, the skin is warm and the peripheral perfusion is good. The problem is one of the circulation meeting a very enlarged vascular bed. In this condition the vascular bed is very responsive to vasoconstrictor-type drugs, and indeed if the situation becomes permanent the receptors become extremely sensitive to such drugs.

There are four other neurological causes for severe hypotension.

a. Simple syncope

This, from the circulatory viewpoint, is a very similar condition. A stimulus arising from the cingulate gyrus (perhaps triggered by an emotional discharge) relays through the hypothalamus, thence through the medial bulbar portion of the reticular formation to the vasomotor centre to produce total inhibition of all vasoconstrictive impulses, and active vasodilatation of the blood vessels of the muscles (Löfving, 1961; Folkow et al., 1965). The sudden expansion of the vas-cular bed is more than the cardiac output can deal with. Venomotor tone falls and the veins become very distended with blood, but the venous return falls sharply. As a result, cardiac output falls while the blood pressure falls to the point of being unable to sustain cerebral perfusion. There is also some vagal activity so that bradycardia deve-lops. With the loss of cerebral perfusion consciousness is lost. The condition is self-limiting, providing the venous return is improved.

There is little evidence—beyond that of anecdotal evidence—that a patient can faint to death. If the coronary vessels are partially occluded with atheroma, the hypotension resulting from simple syncope can precipitate severe cardiac anoxia to the point of ventricular fibrillation. This has been a rare cause of death in dentistry, performed both under local anaesthesia and under a sedation technique.

b. The neurohaemodynamic response

The second neurological cause of profound loss of cardiac output is the neurohaemodynamic response. The neurological pathway of this response is unclear (Maire and Patton, 1956). The effect is a sudden and very violent vasoconstriction especially of the visceral vascular bed. The violent increase in venous return is beyond the capacity of the left ventricle which is pushed into the inefficient part of the Starling curve. Fulminating pulmonary oedema develops (Gamble and Patton, 1956; Robin and Theodore, 1976) leading to profound hypoxaemia, a low cardiac output state, hypotension, acidosis and death. It is a common mechanism of death in the severe acutely brain-damaged patient. It also can occur with brain stem cerebral ischaemia, cerebral hypoxia, cerebral herniation and during surgery on the vertebral artery. Experimentally, it can be prevented by sympathectomy of the visceral organs.

c. Iatrogenic hypotension

The third cause of neurogenic hypertension is iatrogenic and is due to paralysis of the sympathetic outflow from the spinal cord produced by local anaesthetic agents used in spinal or epidural analgesia.

d. Pain

The fourth cause of neurogenic hypotension is severe pain which can produce all the manifestations of shock, hypotension, tachycardia (occasionally bradycardia develops), reduced pulse pressure, low cardiac output, sweating, etc. This situation is most commonly seen in a mismanaged anaesthetic when the analgesia supplied has been inadequate for the patient's needs, but it can develop in patients with very severe pain as occurs in venous gangrene or very severe colic.

HYPOVOLAEMIC SHOCK

This is simply due to lack of blood or circulating blood volume. Haemorrhage and any cause of acute severe dehydration are the only two reasons for this. The response by the body is to increase the total sympathetic drive via the baroreceptor reflexes. The peripheral resistance rises, the heart rate increases, the left ventricular end-diastolic pressure is low and so is the central venous pressure. Expanding the blood volume with crystalloids does confer some benefit. This is because in the intense vasoconstriction all postarteriolar–venuole anastomoses in non-vital organs are opened. Such blood that gets through the narrowed arterioles will then be shunted, carrying with it some oxygen. (Even in the most severe hypovolaemia, the total extraction of oxygen from the blood is not complete and mixed venous blood, although very heavily desaturated, still has some oxygen.) Diluting the blood with crystalloid to expand the blood volume, so that a more normal tissue perfusion results, increases the tissue oxygen extraction rate. It also confers one other benefit: it improves arterial oxygenation. In the lungs is a reserve of blood of several hundred millilitres. During hypovolaemia this reserve is drawn upon. Perfusion then becomes limited to certain portions of the lungs. This increases the physiological dead space—which opposes optimum oxygenation.

Another effect of profound hypovolaemia is the reduced transit time of the red cell through the lungs. Oxygenation of the red cell normally takes about 0·1 s (Roughton, 1952), whereas at rest the red cell transit time across the pulmonary capillary is about 0·7 s (Keele et al., 1982c). With a normal pulmonary perfusion there is a seven- or eightfold reserve of time for the red cell to pick up oxygen. However, the rate of oxygenation varies with the starting point on the saturation curve. At above 75% saturation this rate of reaction is very fast. This is because each molecule of haemoglobin contains four haem groups; each of which can combine with an atom of oxygen. Each of these four combinations has its own rate of reaction, the first three are comparatively sluggish but the last reaction is quick (Nunn, 1981). Thus with very desaturated blood it may take 0·25–0·3 s before the red cell is fully saturated. In the hypovolaemic patient not only does each red cell start at a much lower level of oxygen—which therefore needs additional time for the red cell to combine with the oxygen—but the actual transit time through the pulmonary capillaries is shortened considerably. The net effect is that blood emerging from the lungs may not be fully oxygenated—there is an increase in the apparent shunt effect. Since the Law of Mass Action applies (Staub et al., 1962) increasing the alveolar–pulmonary capillary partial pressure oxygen gradient by getting the patient to breathe an enriched oxygen mixture at least enables the blood to become fully oxygenated. This also accounts for the observation of a reduction in the apparent venous arterial shunt that is seen when a hypovolaemic patient is given supplementary oxygen. Expansion of the circulating blood volume with crystalloids also restores pulmonary perfusion towards its normal pattern of blood distribution within the lungs. It also slows the transit time and reduces the physiological deadspace and therefore improves oxygen uptake. There is a limit; the intravascular osmotic pressure may fall and carry with it the risk of patches of pulmonary oedema, the so-called 'shock lung' syndrome.

More controversial is the role of visceral vasoconstriction in hypovolaemic shock, leading to ischaemic changes in the bowel. Ischaemic colitis with multiple erosions is an occasional feature of vascular patients who develop hypovolaemic shock. Whether these then allow bacterial migration, proliferation and endotoxin production, i.e. the hypovolaemic shock then passes over to a septicaemic shock, has not been fully resolved. Experimentally, this has been shown to be the case in species other than man.

There is a very considerable variation in response to hypovolaemia between the young and the elderly arteriopathic patient. Hypovolaemia in the young will evoke mass sympathetic discharge to sustain the arterial pressure. Hypovolaemic shock then develops late and very abruptly, particularly if the sympathetic drive is suppressed as by the induction of anaesthesia, as can occur in the young severely injured road traffic victim. In contrast, in the elderly arteriopathic patient this sympathetic response is relatively mild. Hypovolaemic hypotension develops very early, irrespective of the state of consciousness and the hypotension is worsened by pain. This is seen vividly in cases of ruptured aortic aneurysms which have not yet discharged blood into the peritoneal cavity.

CARDIOGENIC SHOCK

As its name implies, cardiogenic shock is purely of cardiac origin. Its causes are myocardial infarction, ventricular tachycardia, pulmonary embolism, cardiac tamponade, cardiac trauma (including cardiac surgery) and postcardiac arrest. In all cases the ventricle is at the inefficient part of the Starling curve. Myocardial contractility is depressed, cardiac output falls, there is reduced ventricular ejection and profound hypotension. With the reduced ejection and faced with a continued venous return, the ventricle becomes progressively more stretched and more incompetent. The lungs become more and more hyperaemic as the left atrial pressure rises. (In the case of pulmonary embolism this applies also to the non-obstructed pulmonary vessels, although left atrial pressure is below normal.) More and more arteriovenous anastomoses (shunts) are opened, both in the lungs and in the rest of the body. The reduced cardiac output leads to increased oxygen extraction of what little blood the tissues receive. The venous return is progressively more and more desaturated, and when this passes through the intrapulmonary shunts it adds further to the hypoxaemia. With the falling tissue perfusion, coupled with the hypoxaemia, a metabolic acidosis develops and this further depresses the heart (Tomlin, 1966). Meanwhile, sympathetic nervous system activity is at a maximum. This causes a tachycardia and a marked increase in peripheral vascular resistance. Despite this, the blood pressure is low. If there is coronary artery stenosis, the hypotension may further cause inadequate coronary perfusion and reduced myocardial oxygenation and thus compound the problem. If this is suspected, a limited trial of vasopressors combined with beta-stimulating or positive inotropic drugs, whilst monitoring the pulmonary artery wedge pressure and heart rate, may be of value.

In these circumstances, with its limited or damaged capacity, the heart needs to be as contractile as it can to sustain what little cardiac output it can generate. It therefore needs all the sympathetic drive it can get. Giving sympathetic beta-blocking drugs, even if there are some arrhythmias, is to court disaster.

SEPTICAEMIC SHOCK

Septicaemic shock is the remaining enigma. It can occur where there is obvious sepsis, yet blood cultures are persistently sterile, i.e. the appropriate antibiotic therapy is otherwise containing the sepsis. It can occur in occult sepsis. The prime effect is hypotension—with a wide opening of the postarteriolar–venuole anastomoses—so that, although there is a lowering of the peripheral resistance, there is also an elevation of the mixed venous oxygen tension and a developing metabolic acidosis. The peripheral tissues are warm but pale. Then develops a high output failure with a tachycardia (MacLean et al., 1967). Gradually, the cardiac output falls and the peripheral resistance now rises. The venous return still continues but the central venous pressure now rises. The end-diastolic pressure rises, but there is no response from the heart. There now develops total failure to respond to all sympathetic drive. The blood pressure and cardiac output gradually, slowly sag as the pulse pressure steadily narrows. The metabolic acidosis intensifies, but even when this is corrected it has little effect on the cardiac output. The peripheral arteriolar vasoconstriction then fails; this leads to further hypotension and opening of arteriolar–venuole shunts. The postcapillary sphincter may still remain active, so that a mild tissue oedema develops with loss to the circulation of small proteins, especially albumin, as well as electrolytes and water. Even when these are all corrected, this fails to restore the situation. As the cardiac output falls further, ventilation perfusion inequalities develop within the lung, as in hypovolaemic shock. The blood pressure continues to fall, along with cardiac output and peripheral resistance. The mild tachycardia persists, the pulse pressure becomes imperceptible, while the cerebral perfusion is barely adequate for neuronal survival. Cardiac arrest develops, which is often easy to reverse but just as easily slips back into arrest again.

The only physiological explanation would seem to be failure of the tissues, notably the hardest working tissues, of which the heart is one, to utilize oxygen properly. This has been attributable to poisoning of the mitochondria or the electron transport pathway by some form of endotoxin and hence the recommendation for the use of high doses of steroid, but the results still continue to be disappointing, as are the results from the use of polyvalent gamma globulins.

REFERENCES

Benator S. R., Hewlett A. N. and Nunn J. F. (1973) The use of iso-shunt lines for the control of oxygen therapy. *Br. J. Anaesth.* 45, 711

Berne R. M. (1964) Regulation of coronary blood flow. *Physiol. Rev.* 44, 1

Berne R. M. and Rubio R. (1979) The coronary circulation. In: *Handbook of Physiology: Cardiovascular System,* vol. 1., p. 873. Am. Physiol. Soc., Bethesda, Maryland

Brecher G. A. and Galletti P. M. (1963) Functional anatomy of cardiac pumping. In: *Handbook of Physiology: Circulation,* vol. 2., p. 759. Am. Physiol. Soc., Washington

Brown M. M., Wade J. P. H. and Marshall J. (1985) Fundamental importance of arterial oxygen content in the regulation of cerebral blood flow in man. *Brain* 108, 81

Bullough J. (1959) Intermittent scoline injections. *Br. Med. J.* i, 786

Burton A. C. (1962) Physical principles in circulatory phenomena: The physical equilibria of the heart and blood vessels. In: *Handbook of Physiology: Circulation,* vol. 1., p. 85. Am. Physiol. Soc., Washington

Carson S. A., Chorley G. E., Hamilton F. N. et al. (1965) Variations in cardiac output with acid base changes in the anaesthetized dog. *J. Appl. Physiol.* 20, 948

Dawson P. M. (1943) An historical sketch of the Valsalva experiment. *Bull. Inst. Hist. Med.* 14, 295

Duck F. A., Hodson C. J. and Tomlin P. J. (1974) An oesophageal probe for aortic flow velocity monitoring. *Ultrasound Med. Biol.* 1, 233

Etsten B. and Li T. H. (1962) Current concepts of myocardial function during anaesthesia. *Br. J. Anaesth.* 34, 884

Fieschi C. and Lenzi G. L. (1983) Cerebral blood flow and metabolism in stroke patients. In: *Vascular Disease of the Nervous System.* 2nd edn., p. 101. Editor: Russell R. W. R. Churchill Livingstone, London

Folkow B., Heymans C. and Neil E. (1965) Integrated aspects of cardiovascular regulation. In: *Handbook of Physiology: Circulation,* vol. 3., p. 1787. Am. Physiol. Soc., Washington

Froman C. (1968) Adverse effects of low carbon dioxide tension during mechanical over-ventilation of patients with combined head and chest injuries. *Br. J. Anaesth.* 40, 383

Gamble J. E. and Patton H. D. (1956) Pulmonary oedema and haemorrhage from pre-optic lesions in rats. *Am. J. Physiol.* 172, 623

Ganong W. F. (1983a) Metabolism of cardiac muscle. In: *Review of Medical Physiology*, 11th edn., p. 58. Lange Medical Publications, California

Ganong W. F. (1983b) Arterial and arteriolar circulation. In: *Review of Medical Physiology*, 11th edn., p. 469. Lange Medical Publications, California

Gersch B. J., Hahn C. E. W. and Prys-Roberts C. (1971) Physical criteria for measurement of left ventricular pressure and its first derivative. *Cardiovasc. Res.* 5, 32

Gersch B. J., Prys-Roberts C., Reuben S. R. et al. (1972) Effects of halothane on the interactions between myocardial contractility, aortic impedance and left ventricular performance, 2. *Br. J. Anaesth.* 44, 767

Gleason W. L. and Braunwald E. (1962) Studies on the first derivative of the ventricular pressure pulse in man. *J. Clin. Invest.* 41, 80

Grande F. and Taylor H. L. (1965) Adaptive changes in the heart vessels and patterns of control with chronically high loads. In: *Handbook of Physiology: Circulation*, vol. 3., p. 2615. Am. Physiol. Soc., Washington

Gray T. A., Buckley B. M., Sealey M. et al. (1985) Is calcium important for haemodynamic stability during liver transplantation? *Transplant. Proc. XVII*, 290

Green H. D., Lewis R. N., Nickerson N. D. et al. (1944) Blood flow, peripheral resistance and vascular tonus with observations on the relationship between blood flow and cutaneous temperature. *Am. J. Physiol.* 141, 518

Gregg D. E. and Fisher L. C. (1963) Blood supply to the heart. In: *Handbook of Physiology: Circulation*, vol. 2., p. 1517. Am. Physiol. Soc., Washington

Guyton A. C. (1981a) Cardiac failure. In: *Textbook of Medical Physiology*, 6th edn., p. 312. Saunders, London

Guyton A. C. (1981b) Failure of arterial pressure load to alter cardiac output. In: *Textbook of Medical Physiology*, 6th edn., p. 158 Saunders, London

Guyton A. C. (1981c) Epicardial versus subendocardial blood flow: effect of intramyocardial pressure. In: *Textbook of Medical Physiology*, 6th edn., p. 199. Saunders, London

Ham A. W. (1969a) Capillaries and capillary network. In: *Histology*, 6th edn. p. 596. Lippincott, Toronto

Ham A. W. (1969b) The fine structure of capillaries and venuoles. In: *Histology*, 6th edn., p. 599. Lippincott, Toronto

Ham, A. W. (1969c) Veins. In: *Histology*, 6th edn., p. 602. Lippincott, Toronto

Hardung V. (1962) Propagation of pulse waves in visco-elastic tubings. In: *Handbook of Physiology: Circulation*, vol. 1. p. 107. Am. Physiol. Soc., Washington

Hassan H., Gjessing J. and Tomlin P. J. (1979) Hypercapnia and hyperkalaemia. *Anaesthesia* 34, 897

Heistad D. D. and Kontos H. A. (1983) Cerebral circulation. In: *Handbook of Physiology: Cardiovascular System*, vol. 3., p. 137. Am. Physiol. Soc., Bethesda, Maryland

Heymans C. and Neil E. (1958) The arterial baroreceptors. In: *Reflexogenic Areas of the Cardiovascular System*. p. 26. Churchill, London

Hickey R. F. and Eger E. I. (1981) Circulatory effects of inhaled anaesthetics. In: *Anaesthesia,* vol. 1., p. 331. Editor: Miller R. D. Churchill Livingstone, London

Hill D. W. (1980) Turbulent flow. In: *Physics applied to Anaesthesia,* 4th edn., p. 174. Butterworth, London

Hoffman B. F. and Cranefield P. F. (1960) *Electrophysiology of the Heart.* McGraw-Hill, New York

Jennet B., Gleave J. and Wilson P. (1981) Brain death in three neurosurgical units. *Br. Med. J.* **282**, 533

Kalchthaler T. (1978) The later years: the kidney. In: *Family Medicine: Principles and Practice,* p. 207. Editor: Taylor R. B. Springer-Verlag, New York

Keele C. A., Neil E. and Joels N. (1982a) Circulation through special regions. In: *Samson Wright's Applied Physiology,* 13th edn., p. 145. Oxford University Press, Oxford

Keele C. A., Neil E. and Joels N. (1982b) Heart and circulation: general considerations. In: *Samson Wright's Applied Physiology,* 13th edn., p. 79. Oxford University Press, Oxford

Keele C. A., Neil E. and Joels N. (1982c) Kinetics of the reaction between oxygen and haemoglobin. In: *Samson Wright's Applied Physiology,* 13th edn., p. 186. Oxford University Press, Oxford

Kety S. S. and Schmidt C. F. (1948) The nitrous oxide method for the quantitative determination of cerebral blood flow in man: Theory, procedures and normal values. *J. Clin. Invest.* **27**, 476

Lambertsen C. J. (1980) Effects of excessive pressures of oxygen, nitrogen, helium, carbon dioxide and carbon monoxide. In: *Medical Physiology,* vol. 2., p. 1901. Editor: Mountcastle V. B. Mosby, London

Lee H. A. (1980) Hyperkalaemia. In: *General Anaesthesia,* 4th edn., vol. 2., p. 1597. Editors: Gray T. C., Nunn J. F. and Utting J. E. Butterworth, London

Little R. C. (1981a) Regulation of arterial blood pressure. In: *Physiology of the Heart and Circulation,* 2nd edn., p. 252. Year Book, Chicago

Little R. C. (1981b) Circulation to special areas. In: *Physiology of the Heart and Circulation,* 2nd edn., p. 311. Year Book, Chicago

Little R. C. (1981c) Haemodynamics. In: *Physiology of the Heart and Circulation,* 2nd edn., p 229. Year Book, Chicago

Little R. C. (1981d) Distribution of blood volume in man. In: *Physiology of the Heart and Circulation,* 2nd edn., p. 203. Year Book, Chicago

Löfving B. (1961) Cardiovascular adjustments induced from the rostral cingulate gyrus. *Acta Physiol. Scand.* Suppl. 184

Lown B., Tempte J. V. and Arter W. J. (1973) Ventricular tachyarrhythmias: Clinical aspects. *Circulation* **47**, 1364

McDowall D. G. (1965) The effects of general anaesthetics on cerebral blood flow and cerebral metabolism. *Br. J. Anaesth.* **37**, 236

McHenry L. C., West J. W., Cooper E. S. *et al.* (1974) Cerebral autoregulation in man. *Stroke* **5**, 695

Mackay I. F. S. (1967) The true venous pulse wave, central and peripheral. *Am. Heart J.* **74**, 48

MacLean L. D. (1981) Disseminated intravascular coagulation. In: *Texbook of Surgery,* p. 78. Editor: Sabiston D. C. Saunders, London

MacLean L. D., Mulligan W. G., MacLean A. P. H. et al. (1967) Patterns of septic shock in man—a detailed study of 46 cases. *Ann. Surg.* **166**, 543

Maire F. W. and Patton H. D. (1956) Neural structures involved in the pathogenesis of preoptic pulmonary oedema. *Am. J. Physiol.* **184**, 345

Marchetti G. and Toccardi B. (1967) *International Symposium on the Coronary Circulation and Energetics of the Myocardium.* Karger, Basel

Marshall B. E. and Wollman H. (1980) General anaesthetics. In: *Pharmacological Basis of Therapeutics,* 4th edn., p. 276. Editors: Goodman L. S., Gilman A. G. and Gilman A. Macmillan, London

Marshall B. E. and Wyche M. Q. (1972) Hypoxemia during and after anesthesia. *Anesthesiology* **37**, 178

Mills C. J. and Shillingford P. (1967) A catheter tipped electromagnetic velocity probe and its evaluation. *Cardiovasc. Res.* **1**, 263

Milnor W. R. (1980a) Properties of cardiac tissues. In: *Medical Physiology,* vol. 2., p. 961. Editor: Mountcastle V. B. Mosby, London

Milnor W. R. (1980b) The heart as a pump. In: *Medical Physiology,* vol. 2., p. 998. Editor: Mountcastle V. B. Mosby, London

Milnor W. R. (1980c) The electrocardiogram. In: *Medical Physiology,* vol. 2., p. 1008. Editor: Mountcastle V. B. Mosby, London

Noble M. I., Bowen T. E. and Hefner L. L. (1969) Force velocity relationships of cardiac muscle. Studies by isotonic and quick release methods. *Circ. Res.* **24**, 821

Noble M. I., Trenchard D. and Guz A. (1966) Left ventricular ejection in conscious dogs. Measurement and significance of maximum acceleration of blood from the left ventricle. *Circ. Res.* **19**, 139

Nunn J. F. (ed.) (1981) Diffusion of oxygen within the lungs. In: *Applied Respiratory Physiology,* 2nd edn., p. 404. Butterworth, London

O'Rourke M. F. (1967) Steady and pulsatile energy losses in the systemic circulation under normal conditions and in simulated arterial disease. *Cardiovasc. Res.* **1**, 313

O'Rourke M. F. (ed.) (1982a) Vascular impedance and cardiac function. In: *Arterial Function in Health and Disease,* p. 153. Churchill Livingstone, London

O'Rourke M. F. (ed.) (1982b) Input impedance as a determinant of aortic and left ventricular pressure. In: *Arterial Function in Health and Disease,* p. 162. Churchill Livingstone, London

Parmley W. W. and Talbot L. (1979) Heart as a pump. In: *Handbook of Physiology: Cardiovascular System,* vol. 1., p. 429. Am. Physiol. Soc., Bethesda, Maryland

Pirofsky B. (1953). The determination of blood viscosity by a method based on Poiseuille's law. *J. Clin. Invest.* **32**, 292

Prentice C. R. M. (1981) Disseminated intravascular coagulation. In: *Postgraduate Haematology,* 2nd edn., p. 697. Editors: Hoffbrand A. V. and Lewis S. M. Heinemann Medical, London

Price H. L. and Dripps R. D. (1971) Intravenous anaesthetics. In: *Pharmacological Basis of Therapeutics,* 4th edn., p. 93. Editors: Goodman L. S. G. and Gillman A. G. Macmillan, London

Price H. L., Price M. L. and Morse H. T. (1967) Effects of cyclopropane, halothane and procaine on vasomotor centre in dogs. *Anesthesiology* **26**, 55

Prys-Roberts C., Gersch B. J., Baker A. B. et al. (1972) The effect of halothane on the interactions between myocardial contractility, aortic impedance and left ventricular performance *Br. J. Anaesth.* **44**, 634

Raftery E. B. (1980) Arrythmias and the anaesthetist. In: *General Anaesthesia,* 4th edn., vol. 1., p. 653. Editors: Gray T. C., Nunn J. F. and Utting J. L. Butterworth, London

Reitan J. A., Ty Smith N., Borison V. S. et al. (1972) The cardiac pre-ejection period. A correlate with peak ascending aortic blood flow acceleration. *Anesthesiology* **36**, 76

Robin E. D. and Theodore J. (1976) Speculations on neurogenic pulmonary oedema. *Am. Rev. Resp. Dis.* **113**, 405

Rosenthal T. B. (1948) The effect of temperature on the pH of blood and plasma *in vitro. J. Biol. Chem.* **173**, 25

Rothe C. F. (1983) Venous System: Physiology of the capacitance vessels. In: *Handbook of Physiology: Cardiovascular System,* vol. 3., Part 1, p. 397. Am. Physiol. Soc., Bethesda, Maryland

Roughton F. J. W. (1952) Diffusion and chemical reaction velocity in cylindrical and spherical systems of physiological interest. *Proc. Roy. Soc. B* **140**, 203

Rushmer R. F. (1962) The effect of nerve stimulation and hormones on the heart. In: *Handbook of Physiology: Circulation,* vol. 1., p. 533. Am. Physiol. Soc., Washington

Rushmer R. F., Van Citters R. L. and Franklin D. L. (1962) Shock: A semantic enigma. *Circulation* **26**, 445

Rusy B. F. (1971) Evaluating myocardial contractility. *Anesthesiology* **35**, 328

Sarnoff S. J. (1955) Myocardial contractility as described by ventricular function curves. Observations on Starling's law of the heart. *Physiol. Rev.* **35**, 107

Sarnoff S. J., Braunwald E., Welch G. H. et al. (1958) Haemodynamic determinants of oxygen consumption of the heart with special reference to the time tension index. *Am. J. Physiol.* **192**, 148

Schlant R., Sonnenblick E. H. and Gorlin R. (1982) Physiology of the cardiovascular system. In: *The Heart,* 5th edn., p. 100. Editor: Hurst J. W. McGraw-Hill, New York

Severinghaus J. W. (1966) Blood gas calculator. *J. Appl. Physiol.* **21**, 1105

Siegal S. H. and Sonnenblick E. H. (1963) Isometric time tension relationships as an index of myocardial contractility. *Circ. Res.* **12**, 597

Skovsted P., Price M. L. and Price H. L. (1972) The effects of carbon dioxide on preganglionic sympathetic activity during halothane, methoxyflurane and cycloproprane anaesthesia. *Anesthesiology* **37**, 70

Smith, W. D. A. (1978) A history of nitrous oxide and oxygen anaesthesia. IVE. Henry Hill Hickman in his time. *Br. J. Anaesth.* **50**, 853

Sonnenblick E. H. (1965) Instantaneous force velocity length determinants in the contraction of heart muscle. *Circ. Res.* **16**, 441

Sonnenblick E. H. and Downing S. E. (1963) Afterload as a primary determinant of ventricular performance. *Am. J. Physiol.* **204**, 604

Spencer M. R. and Denison A. B. (1963) Pulsatile blood flow in the vascular system. In: *Handbook of Physiology: Circulation,* vol. 2., p. 849. Am. Physiol. Soc., Washington

56   ANAESTHESIA FOR VASCULAR SURGERY

Starling E. H. (1898) The production and absorption of lymph. In: *Textbook of Physiology*, p. 296. Editor: Schaffer E. A. Macmillan, London

Starling E. H. (1918) *The Linacre Lecture on 'The Law of the Heart'*. Given at Cambridge, 1915. Longmans, London

Staub N. C., Bishop J. M. and Forster R. E. (1962) Importance of diffusion and chemical reaction rates in oxygen uptake in the lung. *J. Appl. Physiol.* 17, 21

Stephenson H. E. (1974) Cerebral anoxia and neurologic sequelae. In: *Cardiac Arrest and Resuscitation*, 4th edn., p. 681. Mosby, London

Streeter D. D. (1979) Gross morphology and fiber geometry of the heart. In: *Handbook of Physiology: Cardiovascular System*, vol. 1., p. 61. Am. Physiol. Soc., Bethesda, Maryland

Stullken E. H., Mild J. H. and Michenfelder J. D. (1977) The non-linear response of cerebral metabolism to low concentrations of halothane, enflurane, isoflurane and thiopental. *Anesthesiology* 46, 28

Sykes M. K. (1963) Venous pressure as a clinical indication of adequacy of transfusion. *Ann. Roy. Coll. Surg.* 33, 185

Thaemert J. C. (1970) Atrioventricular node innervation in ultra structural three dimensions. *Am. J. Anat.* 128, 239

Tomlin P. J. (1966) Quantitative effects of changes in arterial pH and P_{CO_2} upon cardiac output during halothane anaesthesia in dogs. *J. Physiol.* 185, 66P

Tomlin P. J. and Duck F. A. (1975) Transoesophageal aortovelography in man. *Can. Anaesth. Soc. J.* 22, 561

Tomlin P. J., Duck F. A., McNulty M. et al. (1975) A comparison of methods of evaluating myocardial contractility. *Can. Anaesth. Soc. J.* 22, 436

Trautwein W. (1963) Generation and conduction of impulses in the heart as affected by drugs. *Pharmacol. Rev.* 15, 277

Uvarov E. B., Chapman D. R. and Isaacs A. (1973) *Dictionary of Science*, p. 332. Penguin Reference Books, Harmondsworth

Valsalva A. M. (1704) *De aure humana tractatus*. Pisari, Bologna

Van Winkle W. B. and Schwartz A. (1976) Ions and inotropy. *Ann. Rev. Physiol.* 38, 247

Wade O. L. and Bishop J. M. (1962) Distribution of the cardiac output in normal subjects at rest. In: *Cardiac Output and Regional Blood Flow*, p. 90. Blackwell Scientific Publications, Oxford

Walter J. B. and Israel M. S. (1979) Thrombosis in arteries: arteriosclerosis. In: *General Pathology*, 5th edn., p. 496. Churchill Livingstone, London

Warren J. V. (1974) The physiology of the giraffe. *Scient. Am.* 231, 5: 96

Williams P. L. and Warwick R. (1980) The cardiac veins. In: *Gray's Anatomy*, 36th edn., p. 737. Churchill Livingstone, London

Wise C. C., Robinson J. S., Tomlin P. J. et al. (1969) The physiological responses to intermittent methohexitone for conservative dentistry. *Br. Med. J.* i, 540

Zweifach B. W. (1939) Character and distribution of blood capillaries. *Anat. Rec.* 73, 475

CHAPTER 2

Preoperative Assessment

The preoperative visit and evaluation serve two quite distinct purposes. The first is social, in its widest and most humane sense, the second is to determine whether there are any factors which would make the anaesthetist revise his anaesthetic approach (Egbert et al., 1963). Patients undergoing vascular surgery are at greater risk of succumbing to anaesthesia and surgery than many other groups of surgical patients. Apart from the technical surgical risks, these patients are also relatively high medical risks. Many of the patients are only too aware of this. Fortunately, the majority are older and more quiescent emotionally, so that acute anxiety is very rare. Nevertheless, it is an important courtesy that the person responsible for the patient during the operation is able to reassure the patient fully as to the quality of care that will be exercised.

Patients about to undergo vascular surgery are rarely free from the other diseases of ageing, viz. obesity, diabetes, mild renal failure or even senile dementia. In addition, there is more likely to be present other disorders within the circulatory system such as ischaemic heart disease, hypertension, left ventricular hypertrophy and stress, up to and including left ventricular heart failure as well as disorders of cardiac rhythm which can range from bundle branch block up to atrial fibrillation. Furthermore, arterial disease is often (but not invariably) a consequence of cigarette smoking and so it is more likely that those other diseases associated with smoking will also be present such as chronic bronchitis and emphysema or chronic obstructive airways disease.

The choice of operation and indeed the need for surgery depend upon the degree of imperative urgency to relieve pain and suffering, such as severe rest pain or frank gangrene, weighed against the different risk factors. Some of these factors can now be evaluated. In the best of hands, the mortality associated with lower aortic surgery or iliac artery surgery, when there is no other disorder present, is as low as 2%. When there is one other disease present (as coded by the International Classification of Disease), the mortality rate doubles and for each additional disease the risk doubles again. Thus, statistically the mortality associated with elective resection of an aortic aneurysm in a patient with obesity, chronic bronchitis, hypertension, late onset type of diabetes and ischaemic heart disease—a not untypical combination—is approximately 30%. This still means that there is a 2 : 1 probability that the patient will survive the operation.

Patients with ischaemic heart disease and a history of an overt myocardial infarction are particularly at risk from another infarct occurring either during the operation or, more likely, in the postoperative period. This is a consequence of the sticky platelet syndrome: after any operation there is produced a large number of fresh young platelets, which have greater adhesiveness to any roughened surface. If these exist as ulcers on an atheromatous plaque within the coronary vessels and, particularly, if the velocity of the blood flow past the atheromatous plaque is not too fast, then these young sticky platelets will adhere to the ulcer and initiate thrombus formation. There is a strong association between carotid artery disease and coronary artery disease. The average life span of the patient with carotid artery disease after the first ischaemic attack is only 4 years with more than half the deaths due to coronary artery occlusion (Crockard, 1982). In certain centres this risk is taken so seriously that, before embarking on, say carotid endarterectomy, the patients have to undergo coronary angiography followed, if necessary, by coronary artery bypass surgery, before the surgeons are prepared to treat the diseased carotid arteries. Not all will agree with such a radical approach, but the example is quoted to underline the gravity of the risk factors and how they may be considered.

EVALUATION OF THE CIRCULATORY SYSTEM

The first aspect of the preoperative evaluation of immediate concern is the state of the circulation. Apart from the coincidence of unrelated other disease such as valvular disease of the heart, there are five aspects of particular interest to the anaesthetist. These are:

1. Evidence of ischaemic heart disease
2. Hypertension
3. Heart failure
4. Dysrhythmias
5. The state of the radial artery

1. Evidence of ischaemic heart disease

This might be minor, such as a subtle change seen on the electrocardiograph, or can be major, up to attacks of overt angina. Patients presenting with occlusive vascular disease of the lower limbs may not be able to give a clear history of ischaemic heart disease in that the measures they take to minimize the pain of intermittent claudication may prevent the manifestation of angina of effort; in other words, their femoral arteries are just a bit more diseased than their coronary arteries. If the patient has had a recent myocardial infarction, it is worth discussing this with the referring surgeon to see if the operation can be delayed. The risk of a second myocardial infarction is considerably increased if major surgery is performed within six months of the first myocardial infarct (Tarhan et al., 1972; Goldman et al., 1977). Most vascular surgeons are only too aware of this and have made all the allowances that they can. Indeed, the patient's clinical state may preclude any significant delay, particularly if there is a lot of rest pain, or very severe claudication, or the limb is pregangrenous. Nevertheless it is worth discussing the matter with the surgeon, who is in a better position to evaluate the risk of delay. Given the decision that something must be done surgically to help the patient, there is very little difference in the risk factors, where ischaemic heart disease is present, between performing a major operation and a shorter but less effective minor operation, such as a lumbar sympathectomy, but only providing the anaesthetist adjusts his technique so as to avoid any intra-operative hypotension. In such circumstances, the general objective of the anaesthetic technique is to maintain a good blood flow at a reasonable velocity and pressure, and a convenient adjustment would be to replace blood loss with a low molecular weight dextran. In this particular instance, the advantages of improved flow, consequent of a lowered viscosity, would more than offset the disadvantages of a reduced oxygen carrying capacity—but the anaesthetist must know that the problem exists in that particular patient.

2. Hypertension

Over 50% of patients presenting for vascular surgery have a raised blood pressure (Prys-Roberts, 1982). The biggest changes occur in the systolic blood pressure. This, in turn, is predominantly secondary to degenerative changes in the elasticity of the aorta and the loss of the capacitance effects of the upper aorta in storing blood for the diastolic pump that was fully discussed in Chapter 1. The diastolic pressure may also be raised reflecting occlusive changes in the peripheral arterioles. Any arteriole subject to prolonged raised pressure hypertrophies and then undergoes degenerative changes within its media, resulting in a permanently thickened arteriole with a slightly narrowed lumen (Walter and Israel, 1979). A prolonged period of raised systolic pressure which is secondary to degenerative changes within the aorta, will do this, but the resulting diastolic pressure rarely exceeds 100 mmHg. If in any patient the diastolic pressure exceeds this, that patient has pathological hypertension which could be of renal or essential origin. Renal hypertension is not that rare in vascular surgery patients and, in turn, may be due to atheromatous deposits in the renal artery (or both arteries) causing partial occlusion of the renal blood supply (Goldblatt et al., 1934) and a consequential excess production of the various pressor hormones (Tobian, 1962) which produce renal hypertension. Such patients tolerate hypotension during the anaesthetic period very badly. They pass easily into total renal failure, with acute tubular necrosis, necessitating subsequent renal dialysis. A rarer but important variant is if there is significant renal artery atherosclerosis then, just as in the case of partial coronary occlusion, so also they can develop a fresh thrombosis within the renal artery leading to renal infarction. If the patient has only one functioning kidney, the result is disastrous, as severe arterial degenerative disease is a relative contraindication to renal transplantation. Elderly renal transplantation patients have a tenfold increased incidence of succumbing to a coronary death than the normal population and a twentyfold incidence of the risk of a cerebral vascular accident (Wing et al., 1978). This risk is significantly increased if there is already pre-existing arterial disease. Thus, patients with an elevated diastolic pressure may be critically dependent upon the anaesthetist sustaining a high blood pressure during the surgery.

Hypertensive patients are frequently on a plethora of drugs to control their blood pressure. This, in turn, means that their compensatory vasoconstrictive mechanisms are less active and so they are less able to cope with blood loss. Inevitably, these drugs are being taken orally. Gastrointestinal absorption is very variable both in the apprehensive preoperative patient and in the postoperative patient. The half life clearance from the body of some of these drugs is also very variable and may be prolonged, particularly for those drugs being taken only once a day or less frequently. To be fully sure that there is no remaining hypotensive drug in the patient's body may mean stopping his hypotensive therapy for up to a week before operation. This can have a very deleterious effect on the patient in two ways. One rare consequence is that there may be a rebound hypertension, particularly if the patient has been receiving clonidine (Reid et al., 1977), but it can occur with other drugs. In turn, the hypertension may precipitate an intracranial haemorrhage. Another somewhat more common consequence is that the rise in blood pressure increases the myocardial work, which in turn may lead to angina or left ventricular failure, or both.

Since the anaesthetist cannot be sure that all the hypotensive drugs have been eliminated from the patient's body, it is wiser to assume that some residual hypotensive agent is still in the patient. It is indeed better to leave the hypotensive therapy strictly alone and to conduct the anaesthetic on the assumption that these vasoactive drugs are still functioning during the anaesthetic. If, then, during the anaesthetic, it is obvious that the drugs are not functioning, the blood pressure will rise, but this is much easier to control than trying to combat any synergism that may develop between the active hypotensive agent and the anaesthetic drugs.

3. Heart failure

This is more commonly left-sided than right-sided heart failure and is a result of the hypertrophied left ventricle working against an inelastic aorta becoming progressively less and less efficient. Mild degrees of left-sided heart failure are often difficult to detect. Indeed, the only clinical evidence may be a history of a change in sleeping habit, especially of changing to sleeping on two or more pillows at night. Patients with chronic heart failure fatigue more easily than most other patients and a history of recent development of a sense of always feeling tired should alert the anaesthetist as to this possibility. Many of these patients are well prepared for surgery, their heart failure being controlled by diuretics. The clinical significance of chronic heart failure, whether well controlled or not, but worse in the not so well controlled, is the heart's reduced ability to cope with an increase in work load, such as occurs when the aorta is cross-clamped. The physiological objective of medication for heart failure is to reduce the left ventricular end diastolic pressure away from the inefficient portion of the Starling ventricular function curve. Then, if there is an increase in workload, either in preload from over-enthusiastic transfusion or in after-load from cross-clamping the aorta or from the postoperative hypertensive phase, the heart is better able to cope. The alternative is the risk of pulmonary oedema. The patients emerge out of such exacerbated heart failure very, very slowly and, in the meantime, the resulting hypotension, which is the result of this acute episode, can cause further problems, not least of which is myocardial ischaemia and so further reduced myocardial effort.

It is important, therefore, that if the preoperative evaluation suggests that there is an element of heart failure, the anaesthetist avoids any circulatory over-load but is prepared to transfuse blood very rapidly to accommodate changes in the volume capacity of the circulatory bed as, for instance, when the surgeon releases the aortic cross-clamp. Good liaison between anaesthetist and surgeon is particularly important in these patients, at that particular stage of the operation, so that the cross-clamp is removed slowly to match an increase in the rate of blood transfusion, as the expanded vascular bed is filled. In this way, changes in vascular resistance are not too abrupt.

4. Dysrhythmias

There is little that the anaesthetist can do if there is any pre-existing dysrhythmia, except to ensure that it is not intensified by the anaesthetic. Particular care is necessary to ensure that there are no episodes of hypoxia, which can make any dysrhythmia much worse, leading to a reduced cardiac output, hypotension and all the consequences that flow from that. For the same reason hypotension should be eschewed.

5. The state of the radial artery

At the preoperative visit it is worth while examining the state of the patient's radial arteries, as it is likely that arterial cannulation will be performed during anaesthesia. In the patient with occlusive arterial disease, the radial artery is normally somewhat thickened and easy to palpate. This is in sharp contrast to the patient who is to undergo open heart surgery for valvular disease. If the artery is not obviously strong and easy to palpate, it is worth doing the Allen test (Allen, 1929). This tests the patency of the ulna artery. In this test both the radial and ulna arteries are manually occluded, the hand is bleached white and then the pressure over the ulna artery is released. If there is a good ulna artery, the whole hand will become transiently hyperaemic. A poor quality radial artery in a conscious patient with occlusive arterial disease raises the question of atheroma in the brachial or subclavian artery, and there may not be enough residual driving pressure to perfuse the hand slowly through the ulna artery. With modern cannula materials and a good quality radial pulse the patency test is less important as with reasonable care radial artery thrombosis is very unlikely. Wilkins, in a recent review (Wilkins, 1985), has concluded that the Allen test is of poor predictive value because of the high incidence of both false negative and false positive results.

EVALUATION OF THE RESPIRATORY SYSTEM

In contrast to the value of a preoperative assessment of the circulatory system, where the results may indicate the need for significant adjustment of the clincial management of the patient during the anaesthetic period, the results of assessing the status of the respiratory system have relatively little influence on the conduct of the clincial management during anaesthesia, apart from two aspects. These are whether there is any value in delaying the operation in order to improve further the patient's chest condition and whether the inspired oxygen needs to be increased during the anaesthetic. The preoperative assessment of the respiratory system assumes greater significance at the end of the anaesthetic period, in the reversal phase of the anaesthetic and re-establishing normal respiration, and in the subsequent clinical management in the postoperative period. The main theme of the respiratory system evaluation is to determine whether the patient's lungs are in as good a condition as possible prior to surgery and what arrangement will need to be made for the optimum postoperative care.

Emphysema and chronic bronchitis, like occlusive vascular disease, may be precipitated or worsened by cigarette smoking. Such diseases are more common among patients presenting for vascular surgery than among most other types of surgical patients. Another major contribution is atmospheric pollution from burning coal. As a result of legislation, atmospheric pollution from this source has fallen very considerably and, as a result, the number of patients with this combination of diseases has fallen dramatically over the past few years. There is still a legacy among the older vascular patients whose chronic bronchitis started years ago and who have exacerbated their condition by persistent cigarette smoking, although most have now died. Chronic bronchitis though, due to other causes such as the pneumoconioses, is still with us.

Apart from its effect on blood gas exchange, there is another aspect of chronic bronchitis which impinges upon the anaesthetic management. In the absence of heart failure, patients with chronic bronchitis have a slightly raised haematocrit as a result of chronic hypoxaemia. This increases the viscosity of the circulating blood. As an aid to peripheral perfusion through any functioning collaterals, when a major vessel is being clamped off for arterial surgery, it may be worth while diluting the circulating blood with a colloid plasma expander. When reviewing a patient before surgery, this is an aspect to be borne in mind.

In patients with chronic bronchitis and emphysema, the blood gas exchange is impaired. The arterial oxygen tension is low, both on account of this and because of their age (Marshall and Wyche, 1972). In addition, the age effect on arterial oxygen tension is enhanced in patients with arterial disease. During anaesthesia, there occurs an increase in the alveolar–arterial oxygen tension gradient (Nunn, 1964). The net result is that, in patients with severe chronic bronchitis, an inspired oxygen concentration of up to 45–50% may be necessary before 'normal' oxygen tensions are achieved in the arterial blood (De Almeida, 1975). This in turn reduces the amount of inhalational analgesic agent, nitrous oxide, that is available to the patient so that some additional opiate supplement will be necessary. If the patient has been suffering much rest pain which has needed to be treated with narcotics, then during anaesthesia the response to intravenous narcotics may be less than normal, to the point of the patient becoming aware during surgery despite having received all anaesthetic and narcotic drugs in full dosage (Hutter and Tomlin, 1978). At the end of anaesthesia, there may then be difficulties such as establishing normal breathing after reversal of the relaxants. At that stage, too, diffusion hypoxia will be occurring (Fink et al., 1954). This can be overcome by washing out the nitrous oxide with oxygen before allowing air into the lungs. However, if the patient has been relying on a hypoxic drive to maintain normal minute volumes when breathing spontaneously, further difficulties may be anticipated. Hence, when reviewing a patient with vascular disease and who has severe chronic bronchitis and rest pain requiring narcotics, then the anaesthetist should consider whether there will be a need for a short period of artificial ventilation in the immediate postoperative period and to make the appropriate arrangements accordingly. Certainly, enhanced postoperative pulmonary physiotherapy will need to be arranged.

If there is any suspicion of chronic lung disease, then preoperative lung function testing and blood gas analysis are very useful. A preoperative peak flow measurement that is less than 50% of that predicted by the normal nomograms for age and sex (Gjessing and Tomlin, 1972) is strongly suggestive of the likely need for both very intensive postoperative respiratory physiotherapy and possibly artificial ventilation, if there is to be a large surgical abdominal incision. MVV, or maximum voluntary ventilation, although helpful is not so useful unless the patient is breathing normally close to his MVV levels—few are. Patients with large abdominal incisions have lung function test values that are as much as 50% below their preoperative values, even though the postoperative analgesia is effective to the point where, subjectively, the patients do not feel pain. If they have some residual pain, the reduction may be even greater. Hence, an abnormal preoperative lung function test value is a harbinger of potential major respiratory difficulties in the postoperative period.

A raised Pa_{CO_2} and a low Pa_{O_2} are the stigmata of chronic airways disease. Because of the blunting effect on the respiratory centre which chronic carbon dioxide retention produces, such patients can easily slide into mild CO_2 narcosis in the postoperative period, even when the narcotic analgesics are given in conventional doses to relieve postoperative pain. For optimum patient care, patients with clinically obvious chronic obstructive airways disease should have postoperative blood gas analyses performed repetitively as part of their aftercare.

Sputum examination is important. The presence of yellow or yellow-streaked sputum is indicative of active, if low grade, pulmonary infection. If the patient's circulatory disease will allow, the operation should be postponed for a week or so, in order that the patient can be given a short period of very intense treatment to clear the chest infection. This will minimize the risk of a very major chest disorder in the postoperative period.

METABOLIC ASSESSMENT

The third component of the preoperative assessment is the general metabolic status of the patient. Patients presenting for vascular surgery are often obese. This is not too surprising since obesity is associated with high blood fat and cholesterol levels, and among the aetiological factors of atherosclerosis are hyperlipidaemia and high blood cholesterol levels. Obesity in its own right is a source of postoperative respiratory problems, and these need countering. Obesity, though, makes little difference to the intra-operative anaesthetic management of patients undergoing vascular surgery as volatile inhalational agents play, or should play, a very small part in the anaesthetic sequence.

Diabetes is also a common aetiological factor of occlusive vascular disease. Chronic mild slow-onset diabetes is particularly common among patients undergoing vascular surgery. The diabetes is rarely a cause for concern unless the patient is taking insulin. The commoner form of vascular disease among diabetics is small vessel disease, where the patients tend to present for anaesthesia for patches of gangrene or toe amputations. They do also develop occlusive disease of the larger vessels which requires vascular surgery. They can also develop both forms of vascular disease, in which case the outlook following vascular bypass surgery is not particularly good, as the defective vascular run-off reduces the velocity of flow and so predisposes to the graft clotting. Inevitably, this means another anaesthetic and operation which is often performed on an emergency basis.

A rarer complication of diabetes, which has particularly marked implications in anaesthesia for vascular surgery, is the presence of diabetic autonomic neuropathy. This has to be suspected if there is clinical evidence of somatic sensory neuropathy. In these patients, the autonomic reponse to changes in the circulatory bed, circulating blood volume and anaesthetic agents can be very unpredictable. The commonest behaviour pattern is for the patient's circulatory system to respond as a fixed-volume rigid hydraulic system with little flexibility in response to variations in the hydraulic load. These patients are also particularly liable to have significant loss of the sympathetic drive to the myocardium. Parasympathetic dominance then becomes a problem with intense bradycardia, a low cardiac output and severe hypotension. A history of circulatory instability and some degree of sensory neuropathy should alert the anaesthetist that this possibility is a very real one. In these patients, since during anaesthesia the parasympathetic responses are usually undesirable, the anaesthetic should be planned so as to include the possibility of total parasympathetic blockade.

The diabetes in those patients controlled with oral hypoglycaemic agents should not cause any problems, providing the oral hypoglycaemic drugs are withdrawn on the day of surgery. These patients cannot then go into a hypoglycaemic coma, whilst in this type of diabetic patient hyperglycaemic coma is an extremely rare and very slow occurrence, taking days to develop. Patients taking insulin should be managed in the same way as diabetics presenting for any other form of surgery. The insulin should be changed from a more rapidly acting form and given in slightly augmented but divided doses throughout the day of operation, and combined with a glucose infusion. Frequent measurements of the blood sugar should be made, particularly in the postoperative period.

The very brittle, unstable, juvenile forms of diabetes do not often present for vascular surgery—their average life expectation is such that many do not survive long enough to develop occlusive vascular disease which is amenable to surgery. With the slowly improving quality of diabetic control, this group of patients is likely to expand. Occasionally, they can present as a particularly severe problem. This is when salvage surgery is being attempted to save the leg when there is very distal but infected gangrene. The infection makes the diabetic state unstable, requiring increased doses of insulin, the antibiotic cover then reduces the excess diabetic instability to a highly variable but uncontrolled degree, whilst the degree of urgency to treat surgically the area of infection prevents more than a minimal delay of the operation. The risk of rapidly developing either hypoglycaemia or hyperglycaemia is very real. Very frequent and rapid measurements of the blood sugar are necessary to avoid either of these pitfalls. The introduction of very rapid, semi-automatic, but simple devices using specially prepared paper strips for measuring the blood sugar level, has considerably eased the problems of clinical management in these cases. There is a good case for ensuring that all anaesthetists engaged in anaesthetic practices, where there is likely to be a high diabetic load, are fully capable and fluent in performing these measurements accurately and doing such measurements themselves.

A quite distinct area of metabolic concern is the nutritional state of the patient. Whilst obesity is a common problem among patients presenting for surgery for arterial disease, among the very elderly undernutrition may be a problem. Two factors are responsible for this increased incidence in this age group: the obese have not survived, whilst cerebral atherosclerosis and senile dementia have led to a degree of self neglect. This creates two areas of difficulty in terms of clinical management. The first is that the under-nutrition leads to a lowering of the serum albumin levels and this, in turn, materially disturbs the pharmacokinetics of those anaesthetic drugs that are given intravenously—in effect the drugs become, apparently, more potent. The second area of difficulty concerns the postoperative management. Debilitated patients heal badly, develop postoperative respiratory complications more frequently and recover from chest infections much more slowly. Their after-care in the intensive care unit can then become very protracted.

The last component in the preoperative evaluation is the assessment of the patient's physiological age as distinct from his calendar age. Many patients presenting for vascular surgery appear much older than their calendar age would suggest. This difference can be as much as 10 years. Thus a 70-year-old male may be prematurely aged and look like an 80-year-old. This is particularly true if there is much rest pain. More importantly, during the anaesthetic they respond to the various anaesthetic and analgesic drugs according to their physiological age. Unhappily, there is no reliable or objective way of assessing the patient's physiological age; it is purely a matter of clinical experience and judgement.

CLINICAL INVESTIGATIONS

Chest radiography

The value of routine chest radiography prior to surgery has long been a matter of dispute, largely on financial grounds. As far as the patients undergoing vascular surgery are concerned, there are few radiological signs within the lungs, specific to this group of patients, which are of concern to the anaesthetist. Nevertheless, the preoperative chest film provides a baseline for subsequent comparison with any postoperative chest films, particularly if they are taken at the same exposure intensity. The chance finding of unexpected pulmonary pathology is not much different than for other groups of patients, although statistically the probability of finding an unexpected cancer of the lung is fractionally greater than normal because of the common association with cigarette smoking between this condition and vascular occlusive disease.

Of more significance are the circulatory changes that may, on occasion, be observed. These are the findings of small vertical oedema lines in the peripheral parts of the lung fields, particularly of the middle zone, or a filling of the lung fissures, or an enlarged hilar flare—all suggestive of early left ventricular failure. The findings of an enlarged heart particularly either the left ventricle or the left atrium would suggest slightly more pronounced left-sided heart failure.

The observation of an unfolded dilated aorta would suggest that there is a significant degree of intimal degeneration, whilst calcification within the aortic knuckle or aortic valve would indicate a degree of rigidity in response in the circulatory system.

Laboratory tests

1. Biochemistry

The key preoperative biochemical features of concern to the anaesthetist in the vascular group of patients are (a) the serum electrolyte levels, (b) the serum protein levels, and (c) the blood urea or creatinine levels.

 a. The serum electrolyte levels. They are rarely a matter of concern in patients undergoing elective vascular surgery although the serum potassium level should be checked if the patient has been receiving diuretics or has any degree of renal failure. Any hypokalaemia should be treated vigorously.

 b. The serum protein levels. Although most patients presenting for vascular surgery are usually well nourished, often excessively so, a few are under-nourished. This may be particularly so if there is any element of senility. Under-nourishment produces a lowering of the serum protein levels, especially albumin. Since the albumin is intimately involved in drug binding and drug transport within the body, this suggests that the total amount of anaesthetic required to produce light, but stable, anaesthesia may be less than normal. The anaesthetist must therefore be on his guard against producing a relative overdose with his drugs if the serum albumin is low or the patient under-nourished.

 c. The blood urea or creatinine levels. Patients presenting for vascular surgery are usually elderly and in such patients, therefore, some degree of mild renal dysfunction is not uncommon (Kalchthaler, 1978). The only evidence for this might be a high normal or slightly raised creatinine level. The clinical history may only indicate a mild nocturia. The significance of this is that, during major intra-abdominal arterial surgery, the blood supply to the kidneys may be temporarily jeopardized. If there is already pre-existing mild renal impairment, the risk of the patient going into frank renal failure is markedly increased, consequent upon the anaesthesia and/or surgery. The finding of biochemical evidence of chronic renal insufficiency is suggestive that the anaesthetist should ensure that any hypotension is kept to an absolute minimum and that renal function is maintained during anaesthesia. In practice, this means keeping a close eye on the rate of urine production during anaesthesia and being prepared to give a diuretic during the operation if the urine production slackens off. The aetiology of the further impairment of renal function during vascular surgery has been a matter of dispute. If the aorta is to be

PREOPERATIVE ASSESSMENT 69

cross-clamped, the clamp is applied below the origin of the renal arteries. Blood flow in the descending aorta is reduced and, close to the clamp, the flow is only going to the kidneys. The clamp produces considerable turbulence within the aorta at that point. It has been suggested that this turbulence sweeps micro-emboli from the walls of the aorta down the renal arteries. Alternatively, the very turbulence significantly changes renal artery flow (Gamulin et al., 1984). Empirically, it has been observed that maintaining a good urinary output by any means during this particular phase of the surgery minimizes the incidence of subsequent postoperative renal failure and this is particularly so if there is already pre-existing renal dysfunction. It is here that the anaesthetist has a role to play.

2. Haematological investigations

Disorders of haemoglobin concentration or haematocrit are rare in patients presenting for vascular surgery, unless there has been poor nutrition, as in the senile. A specific, but rare and exceptional, group of patients are those with an aortoduodenal fistula. A history of recurrent melenas in a patient with an intra-abdominal aortic graft makes this one of the possible diagnoses. The anaemia that results is simply a matter of blood loss and should be treated as such preoperatively. The importance of this is that patients with vascular disease at some stage during their anaesthetic will be working to their maximum to maintain their oxygen flux (the amount of oxygen entering the aorta each minute). The patient's heart is unlikely to be able to increase the cardiac output further, in order to compensate for the anaemia, particularly if the heart is working against an inelastic aorta with a high impedance, as well as a raised peripheral resistance. The incidence of vascular disease is slightly higher in the patients suffering from polycythaemia. In this group of patients, if the haematocrit is very high at the time of operation, it is worth using protein solutions, such as purified protein fraction or fresh frozen plasma, in the initial stages of any blood replacement. An alternative is to use one of the dextran solutions.

PREOPERATIVE PREPARATION AND PREMEDICATION

Drugs have comparatively little place in the preoperative preparation of the majority of patients who are to undergo vascular surgery under general anaesthesia. These patients are usually very stable emotionally and require little sedation preoperatively, although if they have rest pain they will need narcotic analgesics. Should there be any emotional need, sedatives, tranquillizers or narcotic premedication can be given, providing that due care is exercised over dosage of these drugs. These patients behave, pharmocologically, according to their physiological age and not their calendar age.

It is more important to ban all smoking for at least 24 hours to enable all the residual carbon monoxide that accumulates within the body as a result of smoking to be eliminated. Since haemoglobin preferentially combines with carbon monoxide rather than with oxygen this will improve the uptake of oxygen by the blood. Reducing smoking also reduces the stimulation of the production of endobronchial secretions and so lessens the risk of atelectasis. It is particularly important to avoid giving belladonna derivatives, atropine or hyoscine, to heavy smokers who have a productive cough. The effort, in such patients, of trying to cough up sticky tenacious sputum can provoke cough syncope. It can also produce very severe mechanical stresses on the intracranial vessels. If the patient has an abdominal wound there is also a greater risk of wound dehiscence.

Ideally, all these patients should be ambulant, well hydrated, in good metabolic balance and taking the minimum of drugs that are likely to interact with the anaesthetic agents. They should have been fully evaluated by the physiotherapist with respect to their chest function and any chronic mild lung infection reduced to a minimum.

REFERENCES

Allen E. V. (1929) Thromboangiitis obliterans. Methods of diagnosis of chronic occlusive arterial lesions distal to the wrist with illustrative cases. *Am. J. Med. Sci.* **178**, 237

Crockard H. A. (1982) Intracranial emergencies, trauma and vascular accidents. In: *Essential Surgical Practice*, p. 435. Editors: Cuschieri A., Giles G. R. and Moossa A. R. Wright PSG, Bristol

De Almeida A. J. M. P. (1975) Some effects of inspiratory flow patterns on blood gas exchange in artificial ventilation in anaesthesia. PhD. thesis, University of Birmingham

Egbert L. D., Battit G. E., Turndoff H. et al. (1963) The value of the preoperative visit by an anaesthetist. *JAMA* **185**, 553

Fink R., Carpenter S. L. and Holaday D. A. (1954) Diffusion anoxia during recovery from nitrous oxide/oxygen anesthesia. *Fed. Proc.* **13**, 354

Gamulin Z., Forster A., Morel D. et al. (1984) Effects of infrarenal aortic cross-clamping on renal haemodynamics in humans. *Anesthesiology* **61**, 394

Gjessing J. and Tomlin P. J. (1972) Spirometry studies in patients awaiting surgery. *Acta Anaesth. Scand.* **16**, 103

Goldblatt H., Lynch J., Hanzell R. F. et al. (1934) Studies on experimental hypertension. 1. Production of persistent elevation of raised systolic blood pressure by means of renal ischemia. *J. Exp. Med.* **59**, 347

Goldman L., Caldera D. L., Nassbaum S. R. et al. (1977) Multifactorial index of cardiac risk in non-cardiac surgical procedures. *New Engl. J. Med.* **297**, 845

Hutter C. and Tomlin P. J. (1978) Awareness during anaesthesia. *Br. J. Anaesth.* **50**, 307

Kalchthaler T. (1978) The later years: the kidney. In: *Family Medicine: Principles and Practice*, p. 207. Editor: Taylor R. B. Springer-Verlag, New York

Marshall B. E. and Wyche M. Q. (1972) Hypoxemia during and after anesthesia. *Anesthesiology* **37**, 178

Nunn J. F. (1964) Factors influencing the arterial oxygen tension during halothane anaesthesia with spontaneous respiration. *Br. J. Anaesth.* **36**, 327

Prys-Roberts C. (1982) Hypertension and systemic arterial disease. In: *Medicine for Anaesthetists*, 2nd ed., p 74. Editor: Vickers M. D. Blackwell Scientific, Oxford

Reid J. L., Dargie H. J., Davies D. S. et al. (1977) Clonidine withdrawal in hypertension. Changes in blood pressure and plasma and urinary noradrenaline. *Lancet* **i**, 1171

Tarhan S., Moffet E. A., Taylor W. F. et al. (1972) Myocardial infarction after general anaesthesia. *JAMA* **220**, 1451

Tobian L. (1962) Relationship of the juxtaglomerular apparatus to renin and angiotensin. *Circulation* **25**, 189

Walter J. B. and Israel M. S. (1979) Thrombosis in arteries: arteriosclerosis. In: *General Pathology*, 5th edn., p. 496. Churchill Livingstone, London

Wilkins R. G. (1985) Radial artery cannulation and ischaemic damage: A review. *Anaesthesia* **40**, 896

Wing A. J., Brunner F. P., Brynger H. et al. (1978) Comparative review between dialysis and transplantation. In: *Replacement of Renal Function by Dialysis*, p. 850. Editors: Drukker W., Parsons F. M. and Maher J. F. Martinus & Nijhoff, Boston

CHAPTER 3

Monitoring and its Significance

Few words have had their meaning changed as much as the word 'monitor'. The original Latin derivation is from moneo, monere, moniti (to warn). This meaning has largely been lost. The Shorter Oxford English Dictionary gives no less than nine different meanings: from a school prefect to a large well-armoured lizard (which in olden times was believed to warn of approaching crocodiles), to detectors of contamination, to equipment that verifies television pictures. The current medical usage of the word is to maintain regular surveillance over some medical situation.

It is only when alarm systems are fitted and are operating that the instrument which is being used as a monitor is actually behaving as a true warning device. This point is emphasized, since there are two components to monitoring which are sometimes lost sight of: (a) the maintenance of surveillance and therefore the detection of a departure from any arbitrary but preset standard, and (b) the alerting of the appropriate personnel that a departure from this preset standard has indeed occurred. Many studies, particularly wartime studies, have shown that few people can maintain optimum surveillance of their instruments for more than 2–3 hours at a stretch, for many deterioration sets in after half an hour (Broadbent, 1964). Faced with this problem, inevitably the anaesthetist will resort to periodic sampling of the data, with the real risk that significant events may occur and not be detected. In contrast, it has also been shown, when caring for the acutely ill, that continuous monitoring by machines fitted with alarm limits and displaying in analogue form the relevant signals has resulted in improved morbidity and mortality figures as compared with those following frequent but periodic sampling (Tomlin, 1978). This is particularly true of the patient with a deranged circulatory system.

Monitoring during the anaesthetic management, including the immediate postoperative period, of patients undergoing arterial surgery consists essentially of attention to three physiological systems—the cardiovascular system, the respiratory system and the renal/metabolic system. In the special case of carotid artery surgery, monitoring of the electroencephalograph (EEG) also provides valuable information relative to patient care.

THE CARDIOVASCULAR SYSTEM

The methods of monitoring the cardiovascular system can be either invasive or non-invasive. Although non-invasive techniques are intrinsically safer and less traumatic than invasive techniques and so should be used wherever appropriate, yet for major arterial surgery, when invasive methods are used, the frequency and quality of the signals, as well as the extra information that they contain, make them the preferred technique.

There are five principal parameters in a complete system of monitoring a patient's cardiovascular system. These are:

1. The electrocardiograph (ECG)
2. The arterial blood pressure
3. The central venous pressure
4. The left atrial pressure
5. The cardiac output

Additional parameters that sometimes provide useful information are the left ventricular end-diastolic pressure, the velocity of flow, either from the aortic arch or from a peripheral vessel, or the actual flow through a peripheral vessel. (This latter is more often used by the surgeon to verify his surgical result before closing the surgical wound.) Some of these are mainly of research interest but hold promise of being incorporated into more routine patient care.

There are also several indirect methods of estimating the adequacy of the performance of the circulation. These are arterial and mixed venous blood gas measurements, percutaneous oxygen tension levels (as the cardiac output and/or blood pressure falls during anaesthesia so, also, does the percutaneous oxygen tension, although the relationship is not a simple one), or conjunctival oxygen tension (which is occasionally used to assess cerebral oxygenation and so perfusion during carotid endarterectomy). The rate of urinary production is also a useful indicator of the adequacy of the circulation.

Not every circulatory parameter needs to be measured in every patient. Indeed, it would be inappropriate in certain circumstances, e.g. the measurement of central venous pressure during carotid arterial surgery. Some discretion is necessary. Nevertheless, there are two parameters which are fundamental in the management of all patients undergoing arterial surgery. These are the ECG and the arterial blood pressure.

1. The electrocardiograph (ECG)

Notwithstanding any normal preoperative ECG report, it must be assumed that, if the patient is presenting for vascular reconstruction for degenerative arterial disease, that disease process is or may be affecting his coronary arteries. The patient is more likely to suffer from myocardial ischaemia, if there should develop any hypotension or hypoxaemia, than would be the case in other types of surgical patient.

During anaesthesia, the continuous display from a single lead of the ECG provides three different types of information, viz. the heart rate, cardiac rhythm disturbances and conduction disturbances. More rarely, it may also display severe myocardial ischaemia, if not frank myocardial infarction, occurring during operation (myocardial infarction occurring during operation is much more common in the patients presenting for reconstructive vascular surgery than in all other types of surgical patients).

The patient with arteriopathy, if in sinus rhythm, will have a normal heart rate. Variations in heart rate do occur. Thus the rate will change if there is any disturbance in the balance of the autonomic nervous system's discharge at the sino-atrial node. This balance will be disturbed if the vasomotor centre is disturbed, either because it is responding to signals it is receiving indicating blood loss, pain or awareness, or because the vasomotor centre is depressed by anaesthetic agents. During anaesthesia, blood loss produces a tachycardia. This is usually mild unless the blood loss is severe. The onset of the tachycardiac response to blood loss occurs more readily in moderate blood loss in the elderly than in the young, but if there is very severe blood loss the severity of the tachycardiac response is much greater in the young than in the elderly arteriopathic patient. Awareness also produces a mild tachycardia, although this is usually associated with a rise in blood pressure, lacrimation and a warm, sweaty skin. The cardiovascular responses to awareness are a simple reflection of the increased autonomic activity that this condition provokes. Other causes of general increased autonomic activity, such as carbon dioxide retention or hypoglycaemia (the incidence of diabetes is much higher in the patients with arterial disease than in the normal population), produce a relatively subdued effect in the elderly vascular patient.

Pain is another modality which disturbs the heart rate. The normal reaction to pain during anaesthesia is a tachycardia which varies with the surgeon's activities. The tachycardia is often associated with pallor, but the blood pressure is usually slightly raised. Certain types of pain are well known for producing a parasympathetic or bradycardiac response (Atkinson et al., 1982). The commonest type of pain which causes this is distension of a hollow viscus but it can occur with any general pain. About 10% of young adults during anaesthesia respond to pain in this fashion. With increasing age, the parasympathetic bradycardiac response to pain becomes more common and in the very elderly, is more frequent than the sympathetic response. This parasympathetic response is characterized by a severe vagal discharge producing a very slow heart rate—40 beats per minute is not rare—a low blood pressure and a low cardiac output. The fall in arterial pressure may result in a reduced coronary perfusion, particularly if there are any patches of atheroma in the coronary vessels, so that a high perfusion pressure is normally required to squeeze the blood through the stenosed vessel. Since the venous return, at least in the initial stages, continues unabated, the stroke volume increases. The result is increased stroke work. The subendocardial layers of the myocardium are particularly vulnerable to the combination of increased stroke work and reduced oxygen supply (Guyton, 1981) and may act as foci for ectopic beats which further jeopardize the coronary blood supply. The risk is therefore of acute left ventricular failure or a severe rhythm disorder. The treatment should be directed both at reducing the parasympathetic response and increasing the level of analgesia.

Cardiac rhythm disturbances call for a review of the technique of anaesthesia, with the aim of reducing any precipitating cause, such as the level of any inhalational agent that may be being given, improving if necessary the oxygen supply and checking that there is no possibility of carbon dioxide retention. Other measures include checking that there is no hypotension and, if there is, then correcting this. Arrhythmias that are coupled with a tachycardia indicate an increased sympathetic discharge on the heart for which the cause must be found and treated appropriately. Nevertheless, many patients with arterial disease have arrhythmias normally as part of their diseased state and there is little that the anaesthetist can do, apart from ensuring that the anaesthetic technique is not making matters worse.

Changes in the P–R interval also indicate that the balance of the autonomic nervous system's discharge on the heart has been disturbed. An increased vagal discharge causes prolongation of the P–R interval and this occurs before significant bradycardia has had time to develop. It heralds the onset of bradycardia, hypotension and a reduced cardiac output.

2. The arterial blood pressure

Continuous display of the direct arterial pressure forms an important element in the anaesthetic management for surgery on all the major vessels. These include the aorta, the iliac vessels, the carotids and brachial vessels. It is less important in patients undergoing surgery on the femoral vessels unless there is concomitant overt ischaemic heart disease. Apart from giving accurate information as to the actual systolic and diastolic pressures, the pressure wave signal gives important information as to two other aspects of the clinical management. These are (a) the response of the circulatory system to changes induced by the surgeon in the size of the vascular bed, e.g. when important cross-clamps are applied or released, and is discussed in detail in Chapter 4 and (b) the performance of the heart as a pump (Chapter 1).

The direct arterial pressure is best obtained by percutaneous cannulation of the radial artery at the level of the wrist. In the patient with peripheral vascular disease the radial artery is usually prominent and comparatively thick-walled, and is markedly different from the radial artery in a patient presenting for example, for open heart surgery. The material of the cannula must be sufficiently robust, so that the tip does not split and mushroom as it tries to penetrate the toughened arterial wall. With reasonably fine Teflon cannulas, the Allen test (Allen, 1929) which purports to test the patency of the ulna artery, is unnecessary as the risk of thrombosis or embolization is minimal and there is enough flow around the side of the cannula to supply the resting thenar eminence. The Allen test is not reliable and has a high error rate, with both positive and negative errors, when compared with more sophisticated methods of assessing blood flow, such as those using Doppler probes (Wilkins, 1985).

For cannulation purposes, an alternative to the radial artery is the brachial artery, but this is the artery of last resort. The main problem that can arise from use of the brachial artery is that the position of the artery within the antecubital fossa is highly variable. A particular hazard can arise if the artery lies below the brachial aponeurosis. Any haematoma forming here, as can arise when withdrawing the cannula, can cause complete arterial compression with the threat of distal gangrene or Volkmann's ischaemic contracture. Emergency surgical decompression then becomes necessary. It is essential, therefore, if the brachial artery has been used that particular care is exercised to minimize haematoma formation.

The arterial cannula is then connected, via a reasonably stiff narrow bore tube (this minimizes excessive damping of the pressure wave), to a transducer and the pressure wave displayed on an oscilloscope. Different parts of the pressure wave indicate different things. In the patient with arterial disease the presssure wave sensed at the wrist more accurately reflects the cycle of events which are occurring within the aorta than in the normal young healthy subject. This is because there is loss of some elastic tissue in the aorta and its larger branches and, therefore, loss of some of the damping of the pressure wave that this elastic tissue normally produces.

As seen on the oscilloscope, the arterial pressure wave from a normal subject under anaesthesia consists of a rapidly rising wave, curving sharply to a plateau which then abruptly curves down. Approximately two-thirds of the way down, there is a sudden sharp, small, upwards deflection—the dichrotic notch. Then the arterial pressure wave continues its descent at a progressively slower pace, until it reaches the diastolic pressure whereupon the whole cycle is repeated. Apart from the dichrotic notch, there are no very sharp angles to be seen. (*See Fig.* 3.1A.) The dichrotic notch represents the summation of the changes in pressure, resulting from the major pressure wave within the aorta being reflected back towards the heart from the terminal branches of the arterial tree in the periphery. There is little distortion or damping of the dichrotic notch when sensing at the radial artery, as the sensing catheter is nearer the source of the pressure wave reflection and the reflected pressure wave has not had to pass through a large, mainly elastic, tube. If the dichrotic notch is blurred and without sharp angles, this suggests that the pressure signal is being further damped by the instrumentation. The most likely cause for this is air bubbles in the catheter–transducer system.

In the patient with degenerative arterial disease, in whom the heart is performing well and the cardiac output is good, the situation is somewhat different. The pressure wave travels through the arterial tree very much faster—the more elastic the vascular conducting system, the greater is the damping and the slower the velocity of propagation of the pressure wave. As seen on the oscilloscope, the rising pressure wave is much steeper and there is an initial overshoot of pressure as the less compliant aorta tries to accomodate the increase in pressure and flow that is thrust upon it. Then follows a plateau of pressure which may be rippled slightly. These ripples are minor waves caused by the increased turbulence of blood in the upper aorta. (In normal subjects the zone of turbulence ceases at about the end of the arch of the aorta, whereas in the patient with atheromatous degeneration of the aorta the zone of turbulence extends down the first part of the descending aorta and can reach as far as the level of the diaphragm.) As systole ceases, the pressure wave falls, but there may be two, three or even four dichrotic notches, each progressively smaller than its predecessor, as the pressure wave is being reflected again and again up and down the smaller but stiffer arteries whose loss of elastic tissue is preventing the dampening out of these minor pressure waves. The whole arterial system is reverberating like a bell to the stroke of the systolic ejection wave. (*See Fig.* 3.1B.)

In the patient with degenerative arterial disease a variation of the pressure wave signal is when, at the plateau stage of systolic ejection pressure, the plateau is replaced by a dome of rising pressure which exceeds the initial overshoot. (*See Fig.* 3.1C.) This indicates that the heart is contracting particularly vigorously, that is, it is generating

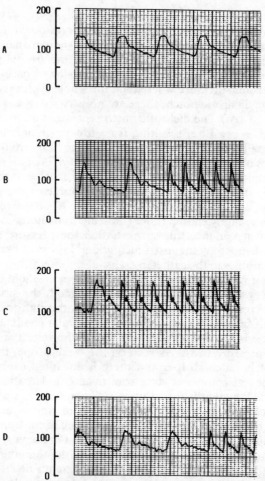

Fig. 3.1. **Blood pressure profiles in anaesthesia. N.B. Note the change in paper speed in tracings B, C and D although the heart rate is essentially unchanged.**

A: From a normal subject. The tracing shows a typical systolic pressure plateau and a single dichrotic notch.

B: This is from a patient with arterial disease. There is a marked initial pressure overshoot and several dichrotic notches.

C: The same patient as B but under sympathetic stimulation. The pressure is high, there is an early systolic overshoot then an attempt to achieve a plateau and the dichrotic notches become more marked.

D: The same patient again, this time with some myocardial depression. The overshoot has disappeared; the rate of rise of pressure is sluggish but the dichrotic notches persist. The sharp angles suggest that the tracing is not being artefactually damped.

(Previously unpublished data.)

further increased pressure despite an open aortic valve and a relatively unobstructed aortic tube; input is exceeding output and run-off. The heart is ejecting blood faster than the major vessels can accommodate. This particular variation is most frequently seen when the surgeon has his cross-clamp on the aorta.

If the stroke volume becomes reduced, usually because the venous return is inadequate as blood loss is exceeding blood replacement, the peak systolic pressure may be maintained, particularly if the aortic cross-clamp is in position, but the duration of the ejection systolic plateau is markedly reduced. The pressure wave descends comparatively slowly. As the discrepancy between the circulating blood volume and size of the vascular bed increases, so the peak systolic pressure falls, although diastolic pressure is relatively well held up. (*See Fig.* 3.1D.)

If the myocardium is failing or is severely hypoxic, the pressure wave changes again. In a failing left ventricle it has been shown experimentally that the maximum rate of rise of pressure (dP/dt_{max}) within the ventricle is reduced (Gleason and Braunwald, 1962). This, in turn, means that the thrust of blood through the aortic valve is less, i.e. acceleration, velocity and peak flow in the first part of the aorta are all reduced. The rate of rise of pressure within the aorta is correspondingly sluggish. More important is the fact that the ability of the failing left ventricle to sustain ejection is much reduced. Systolic ejection time is very shortened. At the radial artery this is seen as a rather slow rising wave, a very short systole and a very rapid fall to the dichrotic notch which in turn is nearer the diastolic pressure level (because the background pressure within the aorta is poorly sustained). The secondary dichrotic notches may be lost as there is not enough energy input to generate them. The whole appearance is one of snatched brief contractions. The appearance of this particular pressure pattern is of major clinical significance as it presages, at a minimum, the onset of a dangerously prolonged period of hypotension, low cardiac output and all the consequences that flow from that.

3. The central venous pressure

In contrast to the arterial pressure signals, the central venous pressure is not nearly so helpful in the management of patients undergoing arterial surgery. This is also in marked contradistinction to when dealing with patients undergoing open heart surgery. The explanation for this lies in the state of the right ventricle and to what extent it is able to follow the Starling mechanism. If the venous return increases, the ventricular end-diastolic pressure increases. If the myocardial fibre has not been chronically over-stretched, as it is in chronic heart failure, the heart responds by contracting more vigorously. This response occurs within one or two heart beats. If the heart is healthy, the efficiency of this response is high, so that the end-diastolic pressure returns to its original level very quickly—and with it the central venous pressure. If there is any element of heart failure, the response is much less efficient, as the heart is on the less propitious portion of the Starling ventricular function curve. In the patient with degenerative vascular disease the main hydraulic stress is on the left ventricle. If there is any question of over-transfusion or an excess venous return, relative to the available arterial bed, the initial effect is on the left ventricle. If this starts to fail, the over-load is thrown on the pulmonary circulation. The pulmonary circulatory bed has a finite capability of accommodating the excess load before the pulmonary arterial resistance rises. Even if this should occur, the right ventricle responds to this increase in after-load by working harder and so maintaining the right ventricular end-diastolic pressure to within reasonably normal limits. Eventually, if the over-load situation is maintained, the central venous pressure will rise. The clinical implication of this is that, if the patient does show a sustained rise in central venous pressure, he is more likely to develop pulmonary oedema than the patient who has chronic right heart failure and is undergoing open heart surgery. These latter patients have developed structural changes in their pulmonary arterioles (Crofton and Douglas, 1981) which help protect the alveolar capillaries from over-load and so pulmonary oedema.

The other end of the spectrum is when the venous return is less than the cardiac output. When this occurs, the central venous pressure will tend to fall. As a result, the end-diastolic pressure falls and the heart contracts less vigorously (myocardial contractility is, *inter alia*, affected by the end-diastolic pressure), ventricular emptying is reduced, thus restoring the end-diastolic pressure towards normal. It is only when the venous return is seriously out of balance with the cardiac output (which, in the meantime, has drawn on the reserve of blood within the pulmonary circulatory bed of approximately half a litre; Wade and Bishop, 1962), does the central venous pressure reflect the inadequacy of blood replacement or any deficiency in the circulating blood volume relative to the size of the circulatory bed. It may take up to 15–20 min before the central venous pressure reflects serious under-transfusion.

Nevertheless, there are two aspects of the central venous pressure which are of interest to the anaesthetist. The first is concerned with normal clinical care. If the aorta has been cross-clamped and is about to be faced with an expanded vascular bed on release of the clamp it is advantageous to over-load the circulation by approximately 0·5 litre—by producing a rise in central venous pressure of about 1 cmH$_2$O just before the clamp is released. There is then an adequate quantity of blood in the central circulation to meet the demand created by the enlarged vascular bed. The second aspect of central venous pressure monitoring which is of interest is the inter-relationship between the central venous pressure and the intrathoracic pressure during artifical ventilation. In the inflationary or inspiratory phase, the pressure within the alveolae rises. This is transmitted to the pulmonary capillaries and thence to the pulmonary artery right ventricle and finally the central venous pressure. The heart responds by contracting more vigorously, but by the time this is achieved the artificial ventilation has cycled to expiration. The intra-alveolar pressure then falls and with it the increase in pulmonary vascular resistance. The heart empties more forcibly, but then adjusts its ejection to meet the reduction in after-load. Meanwhile, the central venous pressure has fallen. There is thus a pronounced respiratory swing in central venous pressure measurements. If the pulmonary vascular bed is not particularly well filled with blood, the increase in intra-alveolar pressure will have little effect on the pulmonary circulation so that the pulmonary vascular resistance, pulmonary artery pressure, right ventricular end-diastolic pressure and central venous pressure will show very little change and hence the respiratory swing will be minimal. Thus, a low normal central venous pressure, with little respiratory swing, is suggestive of under-transfusion.

Conversely, if the pulmonary vascular bed is over-filled and the mean intrathoracic pressure is high, this will be reflected in the end-diastolic pressure and so the central venous pressure, which will show a sustained rise.

There is a happy mean. It has been observed empirically that if the central venous pressure waxes and wanes with the ventilator cycle but the mean central venous pressure is low—less than 5 cmH_2O—the pulmonary vascular bed has been filled to about the right level. Venous return, including any transfusion is matching the cardiac output and there has been no call on the pulmonary vascular volume reserves. This is particularly true if there is little ventilator swing to be seen on the arterial pressure tracing yet there is some ventilator swing on the central venous pressure tracing.

4. The left atrial pressure

The measurement of the left atrial pressure requires very invasive monitoring and some critical cost-benefit consideration is necessary before embarking on this type of monitoring. The technique involves threading a percutaneous balloon catheter through the heart into the periphery of the lungs, where it is wedged into a small branch of the pulmonary artery. During its manipulation, it can precipitate serious dysrhythmias. Once the catheter is wedged into place, the balloon is inflated and the pressure sensed there is the left atrial pressure. Barbiturate induction agents have been shown to produce very sharp increases in intrathoracic blood volume (Etsten and Li, 1955) and left atrial pressure, indicative of transient left ventricular depression. As the ventricle recovers, so the left atrial pressure falls, but recovery is an exponential process and the final last portion of the recovery may take up to 15 min. Thereafter, the left atrial pressure provides a good reflection of the changes in efficiency of the left ventricle as they occur during the anaesthetic period. The left atrial pressure is much more sensitive to changes in the adequacy of the circulating blood volume than is the central venous pressure, due to the fact that the main hydraulic stress of the circulation is borne by the left ventricle. When the patient is being ventilated with large tidal volumes at slow frequencies, the left atrial pressure is subject to large swings as each lung inflation acts as a miniature Valsalva manoeuvre. The left atrial pressure rises as the blood is massaged towards the left side of the heart, only for the atrial pressure to fall sharply near the end of inspiration as the increase in intrathoracic pressure opposes the pulmonary transit of blood from the right ventricle.

In the majority of patients presenting for vascular surgery the information obtainable from the measurement of left atrial pressure can be deduced from critical evaluation of the arterial pressure wave and the heart rate. Rarely, though, the information obtainable may be crucial for optimum patient care, as when the patient has obstructive valve disease or chronic severe left ventricular failure. In such a situation, it is very easy to over-load the left ventricle and the anaesthetist has to balance the venous loading against the demands for a high arterial flow and the ability of the heart to eject blood at high flow rates.

One particular measurement can be inferred from the pulmonary artery wedge pressure and this is the left ventricular end-diastolic pressure. At the end of diastole, the mitral valve is open and there is normally no significant obstruction between the tip of the wedged catheter and the left ventricle. The normal end-diastolic pressure is between 0 and 5 mmHg. Hence, any numerical value of the wedge pressure relies on the accuracy of the reference level of the transducer. In practice, the clinician does not know the spatial location of the tip of the wedged catheter and how it lies in physical relationship with the left ventricle. An arbitrary reference value has to be taken (usually the mean end-diastolic pressure observed from the initial readings) and trend changes from this are used. A rising end-diastolic pressure is taken to mean reduced myocardial contractility. If there is any impediment to left ventricular filling, then the minimum wedge pressure per cardiac cycle, i.e. before the a wave of atrial contraction, no longer reflects the left ventricular end-diastolic pressure.

5. The cardiac output

This is another useful parameter to monitor, although the complexity of measurement renders it highly unlikely to be adopted as a regular clinical procedure. The simplest method is to use the thermal dilution approach, with a rapidly responding thermal sensor incorporated in a left atrial pressure catheter (e.g. a Swann–Ganz catheter). This technique of measurement is prone to systematic errors, which can lead to errors in evaluation of the cardiac output. The principle of the technique is that the bolus of 'cold', i.e. cold saline, is diluted and evenly distributed throughout the blood of the stroke volume and yet no heat exchange occurs between the walls of the heart and pulmonary artery and the blood that is passing through. This assumption is unwarranted in low cardiac output states and the additional heat exchange may lead to an underestimation of the extent of cardiac output depression in such circumstances. This method of measurement is also very technique-sensitive and a crucial aspect, when repeated measurements are made, is that the technical details are repeated exactly for each estimation. Of particular importance is the phasing of the injection with the respiratory cycle and to ensure that the rate of each injection of the bolus of cold saline does not change. Some compensation is also necessary for any partial warming of the cold saline as it sits in the catheter waiting to be discharged into the circulation. The bolus of 'cold' is usually injected into the superior vena cava just before it enters the heart and another assumption is that there is complete mixing of the flows that are coming from the two caval veins—in fact, complete mixing does not take place but there is a certain amount of streaming within the right ventricle (Brecher and Galletti, 1963), which is reflected in the flows through the right and left pulmonary arteries. The calculation of cardiac output is modestly complex and is best left to a dedicated automated computer. This avoids unnecessary distraction to the anaesthetist. Notwithstanding all these criticisms, the thermal dilution technique is a useful, if somewhat esoteric, measurement and, like so much in monitoring, precise values are often less important than trend changes over a period of time. The results of many different studies of cardiac output measurement have shown that they are accurate to within 10%, although repeatability in one patient can be within 2–3%. (Much of this repeatability is due to a repetition of the same sources of bias.)

The major source of variation in cardiac output is variation in anaesthetic technique—thus a deep halothane, large dose of muscle relaxant such as tubocurare plus hyperventilation technique can reduce the cardiac output by 75% or more, whereas a fall of this magnitude of cardiac output from unexpected adverse clinical circumstances and of which the anaesthetist is unaware is very rare. Like other sophisticated methods of monitoring, its contribution to patient care is not very great in the more routine case, but its contribution can be particularly valuable when the normal clinical problem is compounded by multiple pathology of the circulatory system.

DOPPLER MEASUREMENTS

The circulation is a system of a moving liquid containing a suspension of particles and so lends itself to the use of Doppler technique to assess the velocity of flow. In this technique, the extent of the Doppler-shifted frequency of the reflected burst of ultrasound depends upon the velocity of the blood and the cosine of the angle between the direction of the sound wave and the moving stream. It is a non-invasive technique of measurement, so that calibration is impossible without some independent standard, which is usually obtained invasively. Attempts have been made to assess the cardiac output by measuring the Doppler shift of a beam of ultrasound, directed at the ascending aorta at the sternal notch (Light, 1969). Unfortunately, during artificial respiration, the angle of the skin relative to the ascending aorta changes during the cardiac cycle; it is also technically very difficult to maintain a constant angle between the instrument and the skin, without very elaborate holding devices. However, the major disadvantage of this approach is that blood in the ascending aorta is very turbulent and hence there is a wide scatter of velocities. Electronic filtering devices are therefore necessary, as well as sophisticated computer analysis, in order to determine the average forward velocity of the blood in the ascending aorta. Within any one patient there is a correlation between the Doppler-shifted signals and the cardiac output, although the correlation is not outstandingly good. The very complexity of the instrumentation makes it impracticable for regular clinical use.

A variation of this is to use a Doppler probe passed down the oesophagus and directed towards the descending aorta (Duck et al., 1974). This should give an estimate of the velocity of blood in the descending aorta. Blood here normally flows as a bolus (Duck et al., 1974) with all parts of the blood stream flowing at the same speed. However, in the patient with degenerative vascular disease, the zone of turbulence which exists in the arch of the aorta can extend down as far as the level of the diaphragm—whilst the gastric gas bubble prevents the gathering of any useful Doppler information, if the Doppler probe is passed beyond the level of the diaphragm. In normal subjects, the relative size of the diastolic wave (from the dichrotic notch to the start of the next systole) is an index of the peripheral resistance (Tomlin and Duck, 1974). This does not apply when the aorta is cross-clamped. This technique thus has limited usefulness in monitoring patients undergoing vascular surgery.

The third use of Doppler-shifted signals is to monitor the peripheral flow during surgery. The Doppler probe is placed over a very distal artery—usually the dorsalis pedis (Walker, 1982). If a large Doppler shift is heard, it is concluded that the velocity is high and therefore the blood flow is more than adequate for limb survival. No attempt is made at calibration, but the assessment is purely qualitative. This technique is analogous to finger pulse monitoring that is used in less specialized branches of surgery.

INSTRUMENTATION

Whilst technical details of the various devices available are beyond the scope of this book, yet certain general aspects are perhaps worth emphasizing.

ECG monitoring

During vascular surgery the surgeon will inevitably be using the diathermy. This creates two separate problems. The first of these concerns patient safety.

The diathermy functions as a local heat source as a result of the heat generated when a high-frequency alternating current is passed through a narrow zone of moderate electrical resistance. The current density is confined to this narrow zone and the heat produced is a function of the product of the square of current and the resistance. In clinical use, during activation of the diathermy the current will try to find a route to ground. If the ECG machine is electrically grounded, the high frequency current will try to pass through it. At the point of ECG electrode contact, the current is confined to the area of contact provided by the electrode. If this area is very small, the current density will be high and this can cause a nasty diathermy burn. High-frequency alternating currents do not readily pass through large resistors, so that one solution to this problem is to incorporate high value resistors in the ECG leads. If the resistor is at the monitor end of the ECG electrode cable the current will flow up this cable until it reaches the resistor, then when the current alternates it will flow back again. The amount of current will depend upon the capacity of the electrode cable to carry a charge. The greater the ability of the cable to act as a capacitor, the more the current across the skin–electrode junction, the higher the current density per unit area, then the greater is the possibility for the patient to sustain a diathermy burn, particularly if the area of skin contact is small. Placing the resistors at the patient end of the ECG leads reduces the capacitance effect of the cable (Tomlin and Newell, 1975). However, the best solution is to widen the area of skin contact, so that the current density per unit area is below the threshold required to produce a skin burn. ECG electrode contacts should be at least 1 cm² each. Apart from current density the heat produced is a function of the electrical resistance. This can be lowered by using good conducting gel, that is a gel heavily impregnated with salt. When the electrodes are removed, care should be taken to remove this salty gel, otherwise it will dry out. Then, the thick deposit of salt can be a source of unpleasant skin irritation.

What applies to surface electrodes also applies to needle electrodes and subcutaneous wire electrodes although in these cases the unit area resistance is lower than the skin resistance. Nevertheless, in these cases with the contact area being so very small, the current density is high and a subcutaneous burn can result. A variation of this can occur with oesophageal temperature probes. If the probe has a small exposed metal contact, it can act as a grounding lead for the diathermy current or the probe cable can act as a capacitor. Oesophageal burns arising from this source were not unknown in the early days of cardiac surgery.

The other aspect of clinical interest concerning the ECG and the diathermy is the degree of interference of the ECG display on the oscilloscope. Whilst it is possible to use high-frequency filters to block out some of the high-frequency 'noise', the price paid is loss of crispness of the ECG signal, particularly of the QRS complex. It is much more important that the monitor should go back to normal immediately the surgeon releases the diathermy foot switch. Some of the older ECG machines take a number of seconds after each use of the diathermy before a normal ECG signal is displayed on the oscilloscope by which time the surgeon could well be using the diathermy again.

Pressure monitoring

All pressure transducer systems act on the Wheatstone bridge principle with the transducer forming at least one arm of the bridge. The resulting changes in current are instantaneously amplified and displayed on an oscilloscope. With modern A–C amplification there is negligible drift in gain, or in the zero reading, so that complicated hydraulic valves used for repetitive calibration purposes are a thing of the past. Electrical calibration is all that is necessary. This was not so for the old D–C amplifiers.

When the arterial catheter is coupled to the transducer with narrow-bore moderately stiff tubing and a small transducer dome, there is little distortion of the pressure signal and the oscilloscope faithfully displays the actual pressure signal. This can be a source of confusion, particularly if the peak pressure signal is of very short duration and the systoclic pressure is being measured both directly and with an indirect method—such as by means of a sphygmomanometer, or by an oscillotonometer, whether the latter is a mechanical or electrical oscillotonometer. Indirect means of measuring the blood pressure cannot measure accurately very short periods of high pressure. One result of using direct means of measuring blood pressure in the immediate postoperative phase has been to uncover the fact that, following arterial surgery, there is a period of marked hypertension, although the mean arterial pressure is only raised slightly. This is because the duration of very high pressure per cardiac cycle is very short. Anxiety is sometimes expressed as to the risk of rupture of the arterial anastomosis, but this is not a problem in peripheral vascular surgery (in contrast to the case of coronary artery surgery), providing the surge of very high pressure in each cardiac cycle is very brief. Active steps to reduce the arterial pressure only become necessary if the surge of very high pressure is more than momentary.

As far as the technique of arterial cannulation is concerned, its safety has been proved with the passage of time. If small, disposable, non-irritant cannulas are used, e.g. Teflon cannulas, the risk of causing a local endarteritis and thrombosis is very small indeed. Once in place, the cannula should not be disturbed, as there is a slight risk of inducing micro-emboli into the thenar muscles or nail bed, although this risk is vanishingly small. With modern materials, the need for pretesting the patency of the ulna artery with the Allen test is no longer essential, unless there is evidence of ischaemic changes in the upper limb. It should, perhaps, be emphasized that the Allen test is not completely reliable (Wilken, 1985).

For convenience, a multichannel oscilloscopic display and a four-channel pen recorder is the author's preference, using the pen recorder as a trend monitor. Computer programs have now been developed which provide four channels of analogue to digital conversion and trend display with subsequent hard copy output using only a small micro-computer. Developments along these lines, particularly with multiplexing switching arrangements, will allow real-time calculation and monitoring of a number of different parameters, including such respiratory parameters as VD/VT ratios etc., that currently are too laborious and too time distracting for the practising clinician.

RESPIRATORY MONITORING

Compared with circulatory monitoring, respiratory monitoring is relatively neglected. This has been largely an accident of history, in that the various devices that were used for such observations were mainly pneumatic or mechanical (e.g. respirometers, airway pressure gauges etc.) and there has not been the same urgency to transduce the signals to produce electrical impulses. Measurement of gas concentrations has been bedevilled by the cross-interference posed by nitrous oxide. For optimum management, the information from these various sensors requires cross-correlation and computing, e.g. determining if compliance or airways resistance has changed, or if the deadspace volume has changed. More commonly, the clinician does this intuitively. Nevertheless, there are a certain number of parameters which should be checked periodically. These are the tidal volume, the minute volume and the end-inspiratory airway pressure. In addition, if the equipment is available, the inspired oxygen concentration and the expired carbon dioxide concentration should be measured, together with blood gas measurements. If any of these are seen to change during the course of the anaesthetic, a cause should be sought.

Tidal volume

This may be estimated if the patient is being ventilated and the ventilator being used is a minute volume divider. The minute volume can then be read from the rotameters from the anaesthetic machine, and the frequency counted by means of a watch. Otherwise a device such as a respirometer becomes essential. If a respirometer is being used its sensor should be placed at the Y-connection by the patient, otherwise errors due to the compressible volume within the anaesthetic circuit will creep in.

Airway pressure

This is usually measured mechanically by a device within the ventilator. It measures the pressure within the larger airways. It does not measure alveolar pressure, unless the ventilator has an inspiratory hold control or there is a period of no flow or gas movement at the end of inspiration. Normal subjects being ventilated require at least half a second at the end of inspiration before the airway pressure matches the alveolar pressure (Nunn, 1981). If there is significant airway obstruction, this time may be considerably increased. From knowledge of the tidal volume and end-inspiratory airway pressure, the dynamic compliance can be calculated. It rarely changes during anaesthesia for vascular surgery, unless either the muscle relaxant is wearing off or the pulmonary vasculature is dangerously over-loaded. (There is a third transient and trivial cause—the surgical assistant leaning on the chest.) Integration of the deviation from the compliance slope of the inspiratory phase of a pressure–volume loop can enable the airways resistance to be calculated. This is impracticable to do manually, but specific devices are available which can perform this calculation automatically, usually taking their electrical inputs from particular ventilators. These devices are more applicable to the intensive care situation—including the intensive care management of patients who have undergone vascular surgery—than to the intra-operative management of such patients.

Expired carbon dioxide

The use of continuous monitoring of the expired carbon dioxide during vascular surgery is relatively new. From observation of the expired carbon dioxide it has become apparent that there has been a strong tendency to over-ventilate these patients during anaesthesia. This results in a raising of the intrathoracic pressure, actively opposing the venous return, leading to a lowering of the cardiac output and a modest degree of hypotension. This, in turn, leads to increased sympathetic activity in the lightly anaesthetized patient. During anaesthesia in the elderly undergoing prolonged surgery, the minute volume requirements necessary to maintain the end-tidal carbon dioxide concentration at around 4% (4 kPa or approximately 32 mmHg Paco$_2$) may be as low as 3·5–4·5 l/min and, as the operation progresses and the patient cools, so the ventilatory requirements decrease with time. On-line computer calculation, taking the expired tidal volume and the continuous expired carbon dioxide concentration, will enable the deadspace volume and metabolic consumption to be determined. The place for this type of monitoring in anaesthesia has yet to be determined. Continuous recording of the end-tidal carbon dioxide concentration has one practical advantage during anaesthesia. During normal artificial ventilation under some kind of relaxant anaesthesia, the end-tidal carbon dioxide concentration is remarkably stable—to within 0·1%. If the muscle relaxant is starting to wear off, there is an increase in the variation of the end-tidal carbon dioxide concentration—at slow recording speeds the tracing appears to have vertical 'whiskers' corresponding to 0·2–0·3% increments of carbon dioxide. Not every breath will show this. This is presumably due to the increased metabolic activity created by the muscle mass regaining some motor tone. It occurs for up to 5 min before there are overt signs of muscle activity (and complaints from the surgeon!). The appearance of these fine vertical 'whiskers' on the recording is an indication that the patient will need a top-up dose of muscle relaxant within a few minutes.

Blood gas measurements

These provide useful confirmatory evidence that the patient is being well managed during anaesthesia. Since the patient undergoing vascular surgery will more often than not have, for monitoring purposes, an arterial line in situ, the availability of up-to-date blood gas analytical data is purely a question of local organization. If the results of blood gas analysis can be with the clinician within a short time of sampling, they are worth having, otherwise the information is likely to be too old to be clinically useful in the management of any particular patient. The Pa_{CO_2} will give useful confirmation as to the adequacy of the ventilation. The Pa_{O_2} will give information as to the quality of the ventilation. During anaesthesia in the patient undergoing arterial surgery, the normal intra-operative alveolar–arterial oxygen tension gradient is larger than normal (De Almeida, 1975). (In general terms, physiologically, such patients behave as if they are 10 or more years older than their calendar years, bearing in mind that the alveolar–arterial oxygen tension gradient is, among other things, a function of age.) All that is known is that to maintain the Pa_{O_2} to within customary normal levels requires an inspired concentration in excess of 35%, although this, too, is variable and depends upon the choice of anaesthetic technique.

Measurement of the degree of metabolic acidosis, standard bicarbonate or base excess, if the procedure is uneventful, has shown that remarkably little disturbance to acid–base balance occurs, even when the descending aorta is cross-clamped for a considerable period of time (Johnstone et al., 1965). This is presumably a reflection that, during the development of slow occlusive disease, the patient has had time to develop a dense network of collateral vessels supplying the pelvis and lower limbs. There are other factors also. Among these are the perfusion to the liver, bowel and renal vessels is largely undisturbed, which, in turn, means that the blood supply to the most metabolically active tissues is also undisturbed. Another factor is the degree of muscle paralysis produced by the relaxants and the fact that the patient is likely to be somewhat hypothermic. The net result is that it is unusual for a patient to develop a metabolic acidosis of more 2–3 mmol (mEq)/l. In contrast, in emergency vascular surgery, if there has been a degree of circulatory insufficiency, hypotension, reduced cardiac output etc., there is likely to be a marked degree of metabolic acidosis. In these particular patients acid–base monitoring is likely to be of especial importance.

A more recent development is the use of differential oxygen skin electrodes during anaesthesia. In this system of monitoring a reference skin oxygen electrode is placed on the chest and another electrode is placed on the foot of the leg being operated upon. This latter electrode provides good information as to the efficiency of the surgical procedure in restoring the peripheral circulation and as such is of more interest to the surgeon than to the anaesthetist. The oxygen tension measured at the reference skin electrode does vary with the cardiac output and blood pressure and provides a crude but useful minute-to-minute index as to the adequacy of the circulation. The final place for this type of monitoring in routine care of the vascular patient has yet to be established. A variation of this is the ratio between the oxygen tension at the skin and the arterial oxygen tension. Abraham and Ehrlich (1984) have found that this ratio could act as a good predictor as to the adequacy of the circulating blood volume when there has been an unknown blood loss. If there is much vasoconstriction then the cutaneous oxygen tension level should fall. Another variation is the use of conjunctival oxygen electrodes. In this system an oxygen electrode is placed in the conjunctival sac and measures the oxygen tension on the surface of the sclera. The eyeball receives its blood supply from the internal carotid artery, via the ophthalmic artery, and so a fall in conjunctival oxygen tension reflects a fall in intracranial oxygen supply. It is, of course, not affected by cutaneous vasoconstriction and so is not directly affected by changes in body temperature. The conjunctival oxygen tension corresponds to the mean tissue oxygen tension within the sclera. It is not directly related to the arterial oxygen tension, although if the latter should fall then so will also the mean tissue oxygen tension. The main use for this type of monitoring is during carotid endarterctomy.

BODY TEMPERATURE

During anaesthesia the patient slowly cools (Dienes, 1981). Falls in mean body temperature of 2–3 °C are normal, whilst a 5 °C drop is not rare in vascular surgery patients. For this reason, ideally, these patients should be lying on some sort of heated mattress during their operation. The temperature should be measured at two sites at least—the nasopharyngeal or oesophageal temperature will give the core temperature, whilst the skin temperature will indicate the degree of heat transfer away from the core to the rest of the body. Simultaneous measurements have shown that during anaesthesia the patient becomes poikilothermic, with the core temperature falling and the skin temperature rising, until the core–skin gradient narrows to approximately 2 °C. Thereafter, both fall *pari passu* with time. The clinical significance of this, and hence the need to monitor the temperature of these patients, is that the hypothermic cardiac arrest temperature is higher in the elderly atherosclerotic patient than in normal subjects. Even before this, the cardiac output (Tomlin et al., 1966), myocardial contractility and blood pressure all fall with hypothermia, and if any organ has a precarious blood supply due to deposits of atheroma in its feeding vessel, this increases the likelihood of that organ failing. The kidneys are perhaps the most vulnerable in this respect and mild degrees (sometimes not so mild) of renal failure are a not uncommon finding after prolonged anaesthesia for abdominal vascular surgery.

URINE PRODUCTION

Patients undergoing prolonged vascular surgery usually have a urinary catheter inserted before starting the operation. This provides a useful index as to the adequacy of the renal blood flow during anaesthesia. Accurate measurement of the hourly rate of urine production is necessary to detect, and hopefully offset, the development of renal impairment during anaesthesia. This should, therefore, form part of the routine observations made by the anaesthetist during the anaesthetic period.

OTHER MONITORING

Computer-facilitated monitoring systems of the degree of electro-encephalic activity, neuromuscular transmission and electromyography have recently been developed. Their role in the care of patients undergoing major vascular surgery has yet to be evaluated. Of particular promise is the role of electro-encephalic activity in carotid artery surgery. Whether this will displace the more complex true electro-encephalographic type of monitoring used in this branch of surgery remains to be seen. In this respect, the cerebral function monitor has proved to be a disappointment.

REFERENCES

Abraham E. and Ehrlich H. (1984) Conjunctival and trans-cutaneous oxygen monitoring during resuscitation. *Ann. Emerg. Med.* **13**, 287

Allen E. V. (1929) Thromboangiitis obliterans. Methods of diagnosis of occlusive arterial disease distal to the wrist with illustrative cases. *Am. J. Med. Sci.* **178**, 237

Atkinson R. S., Rushman G. B. and Lee J. A. (1982) Vagal reflex mechanisms. In: *Synopsis of Anaesthesia*, 9th edn., p. 819. Wright PSG., Bristol

Brecher G. A. and Galletti P. M. (1963) Functional anatomy of cardiac pumping. In: *Handbook of Physiology: The Circulation*, vol. 2., p. 759. Am. Physiol. Soc., Washington

Broadbent D. E. (1964) Vigilance. *Br. Med. Bull.* **20**, 17

Crofton J. and Douglas A. (ed.) (1981) Vascular pathology in pulmonary hypertension. In: *Respiratory Diseases*, 3rd edn., p. 391. Blackwell Scientific Publications, Oxford

De Almeida A. J. M. P. (1975) Some effects of inspiratory flow patterns on blood gas exchange in artificial ventilation in anaesthesia. PhD thesis, University of Birmingham

Dienes R. S. (1981) Inadvertant hypothermia in the operating room. *J. Plast. Reconstr. Surg.* **67**, 253

Duck F. A., Hodson C. J. and Tomlin P. J. (1974) An oesophageal probe for aortic flow velocity monitoring. *Ultrasound Med. Biol.* **1**, 233

Etsten B. and Li T. H. (1955) Haemodynamic changes during thiopental anaesthesia in humans. Cardiac output, stroke volume, total peripheral resistance and intrathoracic blood volume. *J. Clin. Invest.* **34**, 500

Gleason W. L. and Braunwald E. (1962) Studies on the first derivative of the ventricle pressure pulse in man. *J. Clin. Invest.* **41**, 80

Guyton A. C. (1981) Epicardial versus endocardial blood flow. Effect of intramyocardial pressure. In: *Textbook of Medical Physiology*, 6th edn., p. 299. Saunders, London

Johnstone J. H., Lawson L. T. and Mucklow R. G. (1965) Metabolic changes after aorto-iliac occlusion. *Br. Med. J.* **ii**, 974

Light L. H. (1969) Transcutaneous observations on the velocity in the ascending aorta in man. *J. Physiol.* **204**, 1.P.

Nunn J. F. (ed.) (1981) Time relations of ventilation by increase in mouth pressure. In: *Applied Respiratory Physiology*, 2nd edn., p. 145. Butterworths, London

Tomlin P. J. (1978) Intensive care. A medical audit. *Anaesthesia* **33**, 710

Tomlin P. J. and Duck F. A. (1974) Total peripheral resistance and diastolic blood flow. *Can. Anaesth. Soc. J.* **21**, 482

Tomlin P. J. and Newell J. A. (1975) An unusual diathermy hazard. *Br. Med. J.* **i**, 681

Tomlin P. J., Schlobaum R., Carson S. A. A. et al. (1966) The effects of hypothermia, hypercapnia and pH on cardiac output in the halothane anaesthetized dog. *Br. J. Anaesth.* **38**, 660

Wade O. L. and Bishop J. M. (ed.) (1962) Distribution of cardiac output in normal subjects at rest. In: *Cardiac Output and Regional Blood Flow*, p. 86. Blackwell Scientific Publications, Oxford

Walker W. F. (1982) Vascular disease of the lower limbs. In: *Essential Surgical Practice*, p. 752. Editors: Cuschieri A., Giles G. A. and Moossa A. R. Wright PSG, Bristol

Wilkins R. G. (1985) Radial artery cannulation and ischaemic damage: a review. *Anaesthesia* **40**, 896

CHAPTER 4

Anaesthesia for Elective Aortic Surgery

GENERAL PRINCIPLES

The general objectives of anaesthesia for vascular surgery are:

1. To provide for the relief of pain and the blocking of noxious reflexes which arise from this pain whilst the patient is unconscious during operation and also postoperatively.
2. To ensure the least disturbances to the patient's major physiological systems, notably the cardiovascular system, which are compatible with a good technical result from the surgery.
3. To provide the optimum technical conditions so as to enable the surgeon to perform the operation as best he can.

The first requirement is common to most anaesthetics, yet in the case of vascular surgery failure to meet the first requirement can have particularly serious consequences for the patient and, indeed, can prejudice the successful outcome of the operation. Thus pain, if inadequately controlled, can lead to hypotension, which, in turn, can reduce the velocity of blood flow through a newly inserted graft so that the graft clots, which then requires a Fogarty catheterization and embolectomy and generally imperils limb survival.

It is the second requirement that provides the greatest challenge in the general anaesthetic management of a patient undergoing vascular surgery, as adverse disturbances of the cardiovascular system can seriously jeopardize the outcome of what, otherwise, would have been a good functional result of a well-performed operation. This is but a variation of the old adage: 'The operation was successful but the patient died.' At certain stages of a vascular operation extremely close liaison between anaesthetist and surgeon is essential, more so than in many other branches of anaesthesia and surgery. Good surgical results are the hallmark of good teamwork between the anaesthetist and the surgeon.

Given the successful attainment of the first two objectives, the third is easily achieved with modern intravenous relaxant drugs. The role of inhalational anaesthetic vapours in achieving this objective is negligible, verging on the obsolete.

PAIN: ITS TRANSMISSION,
ITS EFFECTS AND ITS CONTROL

Vascular surgery, particularly on the lower half of the body, entails big extensive incisions through areas of the body well endowed with pain receptors. In the case of surgery on the aorta or on its major branches, this involves the abdominal wall, the anterior and posterior peritoneum and the root of the mesentery, whilst in the case of surgery on the femoral or femoral–popliteal artery and its branches, this involves multiple skin incisions and extensive subcutaneous blunt dissection, both of which are powerful stimuli of pain.

It is essential to block the pain as, otherwise, there will be major disturbances of the autonomic system, and both sympathetic and parasympathetic systems, the ratio of the disturbances of these two subsystems being highly variable between different patients.

The pathways of pain

Pain is a non-quantifiable end-result of a disturbance of a variety of sensory nerve endings. The simplest of these are the naked terminals that lie in the skin and peritoneum, but virtually all other nerve endings are capable of producing pain if stimulated hard enough—even the specialized nerve endings of the special senses such as vision or hearing. Furthermore, those nerve endings which do not produce the actual sense of pain, such as proprioception, are capable of producing all the sequelae of pain. An example of the latter is the progressive and eventual intense distress of being in the knee–elbow position, immobile for a prolonged period of time, with half the body paralysed and insensitive, whilst the surgeon is operating on an intervertebral disc under spinal anaesthesia.

Apart from pain arising from the naked nerve endings, other common nerve endings will produce the sensation and sequelae of pain if those nerve endings are firing at an excessive frequency. Pressure, heat, cold—all will stimulate their respective nerve endings to discharge at an excessive rate so that volleys of impulses arrive at their respective relays faster than the relays can handle them. There will then be recruitment of other relays, and diffusive spillover of the mass discharge of the transmitter substance to cause disturbance of other sensations, e.g. hyperaesthesia.

The impulses that signify pain travel to the spinal cord principally by way of relatively small diameter nerves (those which are more easily blocked by local anaesthetic drugs, but resistant to ischaemic pressure so that pain persists even when motor transmission has ceased as in the tourniqueted limb). These small diameter fibres are incorporated with the major sensory nerve bundles and they synapse in the spinal cord at the segmental level of the dermatome in which they arise. This enables a precise location as to the anatomical site of the pain.

Another important route of the transmission of pain is through the autonomic nerves which contain afferent as well as efferent fibres. All the major blood vessels have accompanying them sympathetic nerves which innervate the vessels and, eventually, end up at the arterioles. Pain signals, usually of ischaemic origin, can travel up this system, but they relay at the same segmental level as the ischaemic dermatome. Pain transmitted by this route is not well localized, but is referred to the general area of the ipsilateral dermatome. If the autonomic pain is excessive, there will be recruitment of other segments, both above and below the segment that subserves the painful area, so that the pain appears diffuse and widespread. This is seen in the vascular patient with rest pain or claudication, who, though experiencing severe pain, cannot localize it more precisely than to a general segmental area that neurologically may encompass several dermatomes. This form of pain is seen in the severe backache of a rapidly distending aortic aneurysm, or the pain in the chest which radiates over several dermatomes in the neck, arm and hand such as occurs with coronary vessel ischaemia. If these afferent sympathetic nerve endings die very slowly, spaced out in time, but progressively with ischaemia, then pain may not be a problem. A dry gangrenous toe or foot is not always particularly painful in the dermatome of the gangrene, but the ischaemic areas adjacent to the gangrene may be very painful. Peripheral neuropathy, notably diabetic polyneuropathy, may also induce atrophy of the afferent sympathetic fibres and produce a relatively painless dry gangrene although if the gangrenous area becomes infected and the inflammation spreads to areas adjacent to the gangrene then severe pain may be felt.

Ischaemia is not the only cause of pain arising in the arteries. Another cause is chemical irritants within the arterial blood stream. In clinical anaesthesia this is seen in two forms. The first results from an inadvertent intra-arterial injection of a test dose of thiopentone, which produces a flash of severe pain in the hand which lasts only a few seconds and then is gone, with no permanent harm done. The second occurs during angiography. Certain radio-opaque dyes, when concentrated and injected under high pressure and in relatively large volumes, cause very considerable pain, which then induces adverse consequences. This is seen both in patients who have been lightly sedated and had the femoral artery cannulated under local anaesthetic block, and in patients whose level of general anaesthesia for the angiography is too light. Although the pain is very transient, it can lead to adverse physiological consequences, such as bradycardia and hypotension. The use of more modern forms of contrast media has significantly ameliorated the problem, but if flow is poor due to poorly definable small vessel run-off, the more modern contrast material will still remain in sufficient concentration to cause some pain. This is particularly seen among the patients with diabetes of late onset, who are undergoing femoral arteriography. Another consequence of the administration of large volumes of hypertonic contrast media in patients with atherosclerosis and diminished myocardial reserve is acute pulmonary oedema (Malins, 1979).

How the pain impulses carried in the autonomic afferents reach the spinal cord at the appropriate segmental level is poorly understood. The sympathetic outflow from the spinal cord ceases at T12. The outflow destined for the lower limbs passes first down the ipsilateral lumbar sympathetic chain. At the lower end of the lumbar chains the chains join together in the midline to pass over the brim of the pelvis into the presacral plexus from which fibres pass to join the internal and common iliac vessels. These fibres accompany the arteries dividing appropriately to supply all the branches (Williams and Warwick, 1980a). Pain impulses arising from the blood vessels travel in the reverse direction. The fibres containing the pain signals pass up to the sympathetic chain and then branch in front of the psoas muscle to join the somatic nerves of the lumbar plexus in order to gain their segmental entry to the spinal cord. It is not clear whether there are also sympathetic afferents which continue up the sympathetic chain to enter the cord at the T10–T12 levels and then descend as a tract to relay at the segmental level corresponding to their respective dermatomes. Lumbar sympathectomy whether performed chemically by an anaesthetist or operatively by a surgeon, can dramatically reduce the severity of ischaemic rest pain arising in a muscle and yet produce no increase in blood flow—apart from a marginal increase in skin blood flow. If the patient is a severe claudicant but without rest pain, the claudication distance may not be improved although the limb may be pinker and warmer peripherally. This effect also is highly variable (Walker, 1982). It is, therefore, important, when asked to perform a chemical sympathectomy, to make no promises as to the outcome.

From the peripheral nerves the pain impulses pass into the spinal cord. The majority of the impulses enter via the dorsal or posterior roots, but recent work has shown that an appreciable minority of pain impulses enter via the ventral or anterior root (Paton and Payne, 1968). Either way, they then pass to the posterior horn of the grey matter to synapse in the substantia gelatinosa. The substantia gelatinosa has been classified by anatomists as having a number of layers or laminae. Pain relays principally in lamina 2 and lamina 5 (Coote and Crawford, 1985). The significance of having two layers separated so widely is obscure. It is unclear whether the different modalities of pain—sharp pain, blunt pain, referred or visceral pain, or vascular pain—are separated on a functional basis or on the size of their supplying axons. In man, there is an indirect suggestion that deep or visceral pain relays at a deeper level than superficial or somatic pain. This arises from the observation that drugs reaching the surface of the spinal cord and which have to diffuse through the cord to have their effect—whether intrathecal opiates, or very dilute local anaesthetics which have already diffused through the dura from an epidural catheter—such drugs block sharp and dull enervating somatic pain better than visceral pain (Gjessing and Tomlin, 1979). Further, when visceral pain is blocked, the block wears off more quickly for visceral pain than for somatic pain.

During the recovery stage, following intrathecal morphine for pain relief after major abdominal surgery, referred pain of abdominal distension or colic may occur even though the abdominal incision above and below the umbilicus can be palpated firmly and painlessly, and yet the para-umbilical portion of the wound is hypersensitive. Then, a few hours later, the entire wound is painful. The implication is that somatic pain is relayed at a more superficial lamina and, therefore, exposed to a higher concentration of the drug as the drug diffuses through the spinal cord. Alternative explanations are (a) that the synapses which relay visceral pain are more robust in withstanding the blocking effects of the narcotic drugs, or (b), that all painful visceral stimuli are interpreted and relayed in their primary sensory modality—pressure, touch, distension etc.—and the conversion to or interpretation of these excessive signals as pain takes place within the brain. Following the use of a spinal narcotic, the brain is exposed to a weaker concentration of opiate than the neurones within the spinal cord. The weaker concentration implies a quicker recovery. The pharmacological evidence is beginning to point to the latter explanation, although judging by the pattern of recovery from the effects of spinal opiates some visceral pain is relayed within the spinal cord. However, this is a rapidly expanding field of knowledge and the evidence is, as yet, by no means complete. This point has been laboured because the clinical significance (of knowing the anatomical position of the relays which are eventually responsible for the perception or transmission of potentially painful impulses) is that neurological impulses are more easily blocked at relay sites than elsewhere in their transmission.

The synaptic relay in the substantia gelatinosa is acted upon by one of the cortico-spinal tracts, whose role is primarily inhibitory. This tract sends inhibitory dendrites to the immediate postsynaptic area of the receiving dendrite (Wall, 1978; Williams and Warwick, 1980b). The mechanism of inhibition is via a chemical transmitter, an endorphin, of which there are several of varying degrees of potency. The action of the endorphin is to raise the threshold of stimulation so that the stimulus from the incoming dendrite is unable to elicit an action potential from its synaptic partner. The receiving cells are well endowed with receptors for endorphin and, therefore, are vulnerable to locally applied opiates (Yaksh, 1981).

From the synapse, fibres pass to a number of quite different destinations. The major flow is via the spinal–cortical tract to relay in the thalamus. However, significant collateral fibres pass also to the respiratory centre and to the vasomotor centre. Visceral pain usually provokes initially a transient breath holding followed by an expiratory grunt, whereas a sudden somatic pain causes an inspiratory gasp. If the pain continues, there is recruitment of costal breathing and a slight inhibition of diaphragmatic breathing, but there is an overall increase in ventilation so that the $P\text{aco}_2$ is lowered. Other brain stem centres, which receive these collateral impulses, are the vasomotor centre and the vomiting centre (intense pain can produce marked nausea). The net effect is a massive autonomic discharge, usually of the sympathetic nervous system, but occasionally the parasympathetic system predominates. Either can cause profound changes in the circulatory system.

Yet other destinations from the spinal cord relay are the ipsilateral anterior horn cells and muscle spindle relay cells, for several segments above and below the level of the sensory input, providing a sharp facilitatory drive to those neurones, so that the response is a substantial increase in muscle tone in all the dermatomes of the limb.

The purpose of this is to provide protection of the limb, by means of muscle splinting, to protect the injured part and promote healing in an animal that is essentially on the move. The endorphins block this response, so that the limb is free to move easily—a clear advantage for an injured animal trying to escape from predators—but at the cost of prejudicing good wound healing. With civilized man there are no predators. The endorphin response is not necessary for survival. The result is pain and muscle splinting or guarding of the painful area. But civilized man can rest and protect the injured part by other means. He does not need to suffer pain to induce him to rest the injured part. Man has not lost the ability to produce the endorphin response, but man needs conditioning or hardening before the response can be evoked when required. This accounts for the observation of the difference in pain experienced, and the shock pain provides, between injuries in battle-seasoned soldiers and similar injuries in civilians (Beecher, 1956) or the professional as compared with the amateur boxer or even the intensity of labour pains in civilized women compared with native women in the bush. An unfortunate by-product of civilization is that civilized man is destined to feel pain acutely, and the more civilized the more acutely.

Yet another destination from the substantia gelatinosa relay is the ipsilateral sympathetic outflow, inhibiting this so as to cause localized vasodilatation in the painful area. This inhibition will over-ride, locally, the normal vasconstrictive–hypertensive sympathetic response to pain elicited from the vasomotor centre, but not the vasomotor response to haemorrhage—which is something often associated with pain.

The principal conduit for pain, though, is the spinothalamic tract. Most of the pain impulses travel up this tract, but *en route* through the brain-stem collaterals are given to the respiratory centre and the vasomotor centre. The main pathway is to the thalamus where it relays mainly in the ventral–posterior nuclei (Coote and Crawford, 1985). From here the impulses are radiated to the whole cerebral cortex and are interpreted as pain and, depending where on the cerebral cortex, evoke local responses, e.g. increased visual awareness, changes of mood, emotion and inhibition of memory. In contrast to the memory of most sensory modalities—pressure, touch, heat, light, colour, sound, music, etc.—it is curious that pain is very rarely remembered as such, only as something unpleasant, perhaps very unpleasant. This is perhaps just as well for the survival of the human race given the severity, in many women, of labour pains. Yet the memory of pain is imprinted somewhere. Thus, when the same severe pain recurs, such as the pain of colic, the intense *déjà vu* of knowing exactly what the next wave of colic will feel like can evoke a profound sense of dread. The opposite can also occur. If the memory of previous postoperative pain is that postoperative pain is not particularly severe and then the patient should have another operation and suffer more severe postoperative pain (perhaps as a consequence of a different method of managing postoperative pain), this can be a source of intense confusion and additional distress.

Apart from the direct pain pathway, there are also other indirect ways of evoking intense pain. Increased visceral activity generates powerful pressure waves within the bowel. These are sensed and transmitted as pressure signals. These signals are relayed within the spinal cord as pressure signals. They are not interpreted as pain until they reach the brain. Intrathecal opiates do not block this pain at the spinal cord level. This has a specific clinical application in anaesthesia. In unpremedicated patients who have received intrathecal morphine during anaesthesia for intra-abdominal surgery, following relaxant reversal with neostigmine, the patients may develop violent colic: pain coming in waves at 3–5-min intervals with easily measurable increases in intraluminal pressure within the bowel. (*See Fig. 4.1.*) The pain is referred to T10. Yet above and below this segmental level the surgical wound of, say, an aortic aneurysmectomy can be very firmly palpated without causing pain, i.e. there is a good somatic analgesia. If the operation has lasted more than 3 hours, it is unlikely

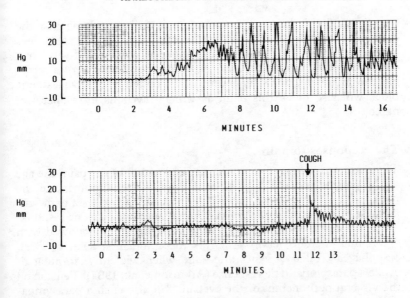

RECTAL   PRESSURES

Fig. 4.1. **The effect of neostigmine on intraluminal rectal pressure. The upper tracing is from a patient who had had no premedication or subcutaneous
atropine. Three minutes after the administration of neostigmine the rectal
pressure rose, then large colic-type waves appeared at minute intervals.
These eventually did settle to larger waves occurring at up to 5-min intervals.
The lower tracing is from a patient who had been given atropine 0·6 mg subcutaneously 2 hours earlier. Note that there is negligible effect on rectal pressure even though a cough will evoke a transient rise in pressure. Both
patients had had femoral popliteal by-pass surgery and the anaesthesia for
both consisted of intrathecal morphine, nitrous oxide and enflurane (0·5%),
and muscle relaxants. Reversal consisted of atropine 1·2 mg i.v. followed 3
min later by neostigmine 5·0 mg.**
(Previously unpublished data.)

that the patient will feel this colic as, presumably, enough of the
intrathecal opiate has diffused through the foramen magnum to exert
its effect on the brain. Oddly, this particular pain problem seems to be
related only to those patients who have had an intraperitoneal
operation. Resection of an aortic aneurysm, aorto-iliac surgery, or
even the common cholecystectomy, all can evoke this pain problem,
yet it does not occur after haemorrhoidectomy or carotid artery
surgery, or thoracic surgery. Premedication with subcutaneous atropine or subcutaneous atropine at induction of anaesthesia will block
this response, although intravenous atropine will not. Intravenous
atropine does not stay in the circulation long enough to have any
significant effect on bowel motility. The atropine must stay in the

circulation for at least an hour before it will protect against the excessive peristalsis produced by neostigmine. If this colic does occur, intravenous pethidine will relieve it more effectively than either morphine or diamorphine. Blocking the afferent nerves carrying the pressure signals by means of an epidural local anaesthetic block will also block this pain, as will intravenous intra-operative narcotics.

The responses to pain

These are varied according to the site and nature of the pain, the age of the patient and the physical and emotional environment of the patient. Thus stretching the cervical os usually provokes a parasympathetic response under light anaesthesia, but a sympathetic response in the labouring woman. Pain arising from areas well endowed with autonomic afferent nerves—such as the sphincters, anal, cervical, oesophageal, biliary, pancreatic—all, when violently stimulated, evoke a parasympathetic response (Atkinson et al., 1982). Tension on the visceral peritoneum, or the eyeball, will also elicit a parasympathetic response of bradycardia, hypotension, reduced stroke volume, reduced cardiac output, reduced venous return and lacrimation. A small peripheral compensatory sympathetic discharge will also be elicited consisting of peripheral vasoconstriction and sweating, but the dominant circulatory response is a parasympathetic one. Pain arising from a somatic area usually provokes a sympathetic response principally of a tachycardia, raised cardiac output and hypertension and eventually sweating. Such a response is seen on skin incision (and sometimes during skin closure) or during blunt dissection. In young subjects, below the age of 40, the response to somatic pain in 90% of patients is a sympathetic one; the remainder exhibit a parasympathetic response to pain. With increasing age the proportion of patients showing a parasympathetic response to pain gradually increases. In older subjects, and particularly in elderly vascular patients, the response to a painful somatic stimulus is more likely to be a parasympathetic one than a sympathetic one, e.g. this response is often seen during the subcutaneous tunnelling of an axillo-femoral bypass graft.

If the pain is severe and prolonged, the loss of circulating fluid volume, in part from sweating but mainly from the increased capillary permeability induced by the increased output of circulating adrenaline, can induce marked dehydration and eventually circulatory collapse, with tachycardia and hypotension. This particular response rarely, if ever, occurs during anaesthesia, but may be seen preoperatively in patients with simultaneous arterial and venous gangrene, as in Buerger's disease.

Another and quite distinct response to pain is hypoxaemia. All

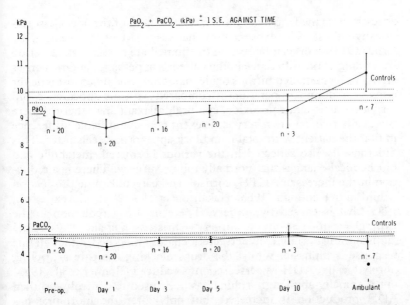

Fig. 4.2. **The effect of pain on Pa_{O_2} and Pa_{CO_2}. Twenty elderly patients, all with fractured neck of femur, had blood gases measured both preoperatively and then postoperatively until the patients were ambulant. The horizontal line is the control line from patients of the same age but not in pain. Note the hypoxaemia did not improve until the patients were free from all pain and were ambulant.**
(From Phillips G. and Tomlin P. J., unpublished data.)

severe pain induces hypoxaemia, via a disturbance of the ventilation perfusion ratio. This hypoxaemia occurs after all forms of surgery. It is considerably ameliorated by intrathecal or epidural narcotics and returns when the epidural narcotic wears off. Even when the painful area is well away from any respiratory movement, e.g. after hip joint surgery, there is marked hypoxaemia. The hypoxaemia is associated with a mild tachypnoea so that the Pa_{CO_2} is lowered. This hypoxaemia is also seen in patients with painful conditions prior to surgery, e.g. fractured necks of femur (*Fig.* 4.2). The hypoxaemia by itself is not particularly severe but it is additional to the hypoxaemia associated with age (Phillips and Tomlin, 1977). Details of the controlling mechanism of this hypoxaemia are not known, nor is its physiological significance or purpose.

There is little doubt that pain can produce adverse physiological consequences, even when the cerebral cortex has been supplied with narcotics to the point where the patient is not consciously aware of pain and is well into the postoperative period. Similar adverse consequences also occur during anaesthesia when the quality of the anaesthetic is inadequate. This is a re-statement of the anoci-association hypothesis first expressed in the early part of this century by Crile (1913). This can be seen in the immediate postoperative period by looking at the difference in the patient's appearance and responses after a well conducted nitrous oxide, narcotic, relaxant anaesthetic for a major abdominal operation as compared with his appearance and responses after a nitrous oxide, epidural, relaxant anaesthetic. There is a qualitative, and to a very large exent non-quantifiable, difference in that the patient with total pain block appears and feels fitter. This difference is also reflected in the various hormonal, metabolic and biochemical changes that normally follow surgery. There is a reduction in the increased ACTH, cortisol, and catecholamine production (Child and Kaufman, 1985; Hakanson et al., 1985; Hjortso et al., 1985) that is caused by surgery. There is also a reduction in the hyperglycaemic response to surgery (Christensen et al., 1982). ADH (anti-diuretic hormone) hypersecretion is also modified, although this response is biphasic. Whilst the drugs blocking the pain are acting purely locally, ADH hypersecretion is reduced (Bonnet et al., 1982) but if spinally applied morphine has been used to control pain then ADH production is increased, but only after the morphine has diffused upwards to reach the brain (Korinek et al., 1985). This second effect is due to the direct action of morphine on the brain. Patients who have had their pain controlled below the level of the cerebral peduncles are in a better condition than those whose pain has been controlled by drugs acting on the thalamus, hypothalamus and higher centres within the brain. This appearance of well-being can create a mild euphoria particularly among any ill-informed attendants or visitors, however the well-being only lasts whilst the analgesia is acting at the spinal cord level.

Pain control

There are three distinct methods of controlling pain during and after vascular surgery. These are:

1. Intravenous analgesics
2. The use of local anaesthetic agents
3. The use of spinal opiates

1. Intravenous analgesics

The simplest method of controlling pain is the use of intravenous narcotics. Intravenous analgesics can be given either as bolus doses or by continuous slow infusion by some form of pump (Church, 1979;

Welchew, 1983). Continuous infusion of a narcotic avoids the problem of recurrent pain as occurs when the bolus dose wears off, but it requires expensive complex equipment, complete with over-riding safety circuits as well as alarm circuits, to prevent accidental over-infusion from instrumental malfunction. During operation, unless the surgery is extremely protracted, there is little to choose between periodic bolus doses and continuous intravenous infusion. Postoperatively the situation is different. In order to avoid accidental insidious, cumulative over-dosage, the rate of infusion must be titrated against the patient's pain. Since postoperative pain is cyclical, waxing and waning periodically over an increasingly lengthening time-base (Gjessing and Tomlin, 1979), this requires that the rate of infusion should be frequently adjusted if total pain control is to be achieved. This, in turn, requires that the quality of supervision must be of a very high calibre. In practice, this is rarely achieved, although the quality of pain control obtained by continuous intravenous infusion of narcotics is significantly superior to that obtained by periodic intramuscular injections of narcotics. The choice of intravenous analgesic lies between pethidine, morphine (or papaveretum), diamorphine, phenoperidine and fentanyl.

Pethidine is not a particularly powerful analgesic and it does, in quite a high proportion of patients, cause a marked hypotension. If used postoperatively, there is one other difficulty. Pethidine also has a ceiling effect whereby, if the pain is very severe, additional doses produce disorientation and depression of the major physiological systems without fully controlling the pain.

Intravenous morphine (or diamorphine) has no ceiling effect as far as analgesia is concerned. Its principal advantages are that it has little effect on the circulation—although if the vasomotor centre is working hard to sustain some level of blood pressure, the general sedative properties of morphine will depress the hyperactive vasomotor centre and so a hypotension will result. Its disadvantages are that it is a powerful respiratory depressant and it is very slow in onset of action—up to 15 min after intravenous administration. Its half-life after intravenous injection is between 2 and 3 hours (Pharmaceutical Codex, 1979a), that is, its duration of action is somewhat variable. In the United Kingdom the bacteriostatic preservatives in which it is dissolved are marginally toxic (Mathews, 1977). In the United States of America, the preservatives used there are non-toxic and this has led to the use of heroic doses of morphine intra-operatively for such procedures as open heart surgery (Hasbrouk, 1970). Such techniques should only be used if the patient is to be admitted to an intensive care unit at the end of surgery. Postoperatively, morphine's euphoriant action and time-telescoping action are undoubtedly advantageous, but its disadvantages are its respiratory depressant action, the fact that it inhibits the recovery of normal bowel activity and that it is a powerful emetic. If very large doses are used, the respiratory depressant effects may also involve the laryngeal protective reflexes. If, then, emesis does occur the patient is at risk of inhalation of the stomach contents with all the problems that this involves. In this respect over-dosage of morphine is not unlike overdose of alcohol.

Fentanyl is an even more powerful respiratory depressant and its onset time of action is very short. Its duration of action is also very short and somewhat abrupt. The initial reports that its duration of action was less than 15 min are now being seriously challenged. It causes very little disturbance to the circulation. Because of its analgesic potency and the speed with which the patient descends into deep analgesia and then recovers from this depth very quickly, only small amounts need to be given at any one time, and this does lead to a somewhat swinging anaesthetic although if the drug is given by a constant infusion pump these swings can be evened out. The addition of droperidol also helps to even out these swings. Fentanyl does accumulate in the body fat and this has raised the possibility that if the cumulative dose given is large there might be some delayed reactivation and mobilization from the body fat depots in the post-operative period. Fentanyl is too potent an analgesic and too powerful a respiratory depressant to be used in the postoperative period by nursing staff.

Phenoperidine is a much milder form of fentanyl. Like fentanyl it is very quick in onset, but its duration of action, approximately 1 hour, is much more predictable. Its analgesic potency and duration of action are both potentiated by droperidol, although the latter is a feeble adrenergic alpha-receptor blocker and so may cause some hypotension. It is a respiratory depressant but not so powerfully so as fentanyl. Its short duration of action, 1 hour compared with 4–6 hours for morphine, makes it unsuitable for use for routine post-operative analgesia.

2. The use of local anaesthetic agents

The only effective way of obtaining good analgesia with local anaes-thetic agents, in vascular surgery, is to use either a spinal or an epidural block. After due allowance has been made for their indivi-dual pharmacokinetic properties, the choice of local anaesthetic drug is immaterial. However, both spinal and epidural analgesics produce severe hypotension which the arteriopathic patient cannot withstand. Although the blood pressure can be restored by the use of vasocon-strictor drugs, some of these also cause venuole vasoconstriction leading to mild peripheral oedema and some loss of circulating blood volume. The velocity of flow through a graft, e.g. an ileo–popliteal graft, would appear to be somewhat slower following epidural block and some would maintain that this leads to a greater incidence of graft thrombosis. However, it is the coronary perfusion that is at greatest risk and the arteriosclerotic hypertensive patient appears to withstand any form of epidural block very badly.

There is one other practical aspect. These patients are elderly and often have marked spinal osteo-arthritis. The various foramina in the spinal canal are often more narrowed than normal. This can lead to a somewhat unpredictable spread of the epidural block which may extend higher than was anticipated. Technically, this osteo-arthritis can make insertion of an epidural catheter somewhat difficult. Apart from the narrower joint spaces the rigidity and denseness of the various spinal ligaments make epidural catheterization, in the elderly arteriosclerotic patient, markedly more difficult and more hazardous (inadvertent dural tap or subdural bleeding) than in the more conventional maternity epidural case. This situation is unique in being the one where blunt needles are more advantageous than sharp needles.

The principal disadvantage of the use of spinally applied local analgesics is the interference that they produce on the vasomotor system. In the anaesthetic management of patients undergoing arterial surgery, there is a need for a rapidly acting and rapidly responding vasomotor system to make the appropriate circulatory adjustments, when the size of the vascular bed or circulating blood volume is materially changed. By blocking the lower portion of the sympathetic outflow of the spinal cord the spinally applied local analgesics materially disturb the responsiveness of this system.

3. The use of spinal opiates

The introduction of spinal opiates into clinical practice (Wang et al., 1979) has revolutionized the analgesic care of vascular patients. The choice lies between epidural and intrathecal opiates. Epidural opiates in the elderly arteriopathic patient behave essentially as slow intrathecal narcotics. Commonly, the blood supply within the spinal canal in these patients is somewhat sparse. This means that there is very little immediate systemic absorption of the narcotic. The analgesic diffuses through the spinal meninges to reach the dorsal horns and the substantia gelatinosa. The duration of action of a single dose of epidural morphine in these patients is approximately 24 hours. The analgesic onset time of epidural morphine in these patients is approximately 30–45 min (Camporesi and Redick, 1983). This is too slow to be the principal analgesic for surgery, and the temptation has been to use a local anaesthetic epidural block as a starter, with all the difficulties which attend that technique. Postoperatively epidural morphine has distinct advantages, not least is that it can be topped up once daily to cover the expected 5 days of marked postoperative pain which follow resection of an abdominal aortic aneurysm. Meningeal absorption starts immediately, but it is a very slow process in these elderly patients and there is also some slow systemic absorption of the narcotic. Eventually 30–50% of the epidural narcotic may be absorbed systemically. In the young patient with a hyperaemic epidural space there may be as much as 100% systemic absorption (Husemeyer et al., 1980). In the elderly patient the systemic absorption is simply countered by giving a slightly larger dose of narcotic. Rarely, but sufficiently frequently to be disturbing, the whole epidural dose transfers comparatively rapidly into the subarachnoid space to produce severe, delayed and unexpected respiratory depression (Scott and McClure, 1979) identical to that following an overdose of intrathecal narcotic. This can occur even when there has been a prior local anaesthetic through the same epidural catheter, which has produced a normal epidural block.

Intrathecal narcotics such as morphine behave in a much more predictable fashion. The onset of analgesia is 3–10 min, the duration is somewhat variable but ranges from 1 to 4 days. The speed of onset of action makes intrathecal morphine suitable for use during surgery, providing that the patient's condition allows for the manhandling and changes of posture that accompany lumbar puncture immediately following induction of anaesthesia. Because of its potency and long duration of action, no other analgesic is necessary during anaesthesia (although sleep must be ensured by independent means). Haemodynamic stability is substantial and is subject only to those changes produced by the surgery. There appears to be no interaction with any other drug. However, the chief advantage lies in the quality and duration of postoperative analgesia. Duration of analgesia is somewhat difficult to determine as severe postoperative pain, after many operations, lasts less than 3 days. However, after abdominal aortic aneurysmectomy severe pain lasts not less than 4 days. This has enabled a more accurate identification of the duration of action of intrathecal morphine (*Fig.* 4.3). As might be expected, the pattern of duration follows a typical sigmoid response curve. Morphine has been the drug most studied although diamorphine (Kaufman, 1981), pethidine (Cousins et al., 1977), fentanyl and buprenorphine (Srivastava, 1982) have all been tried. The duration of action of these narcotics, when given intrathecally, is appreciably less than that of morphine.

For the vascular patient the ideal dose of intrathecal morphine lies between 0·5 and 1·4 mg depending upon the patient's age, body length and site of operation—body weight is immaterial as the drug is confined to within the theca (Gjessing and Tomlin, 1981). Increasing

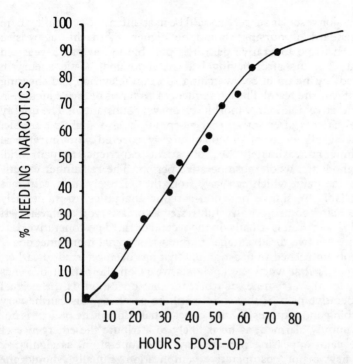

Fig. 4.3. **Duration of analgesia after intrathecal morphine. The median time was 36 hours before the patient required any analgesic postoperatively. Approximately 10 % of patients did not require any additional analgesic during the whole of their postoperative period. Data from 14 patients all of whom had undergone surgery on the infra-renal portion of the aorta.** (Previously unpublished data.)

the dose beyond the optimum leads to a prolongation of the analgesia but a very much higher risk of delayed respiratory depression. Following a normal dose of intrathecal morphine, and given reasonable nursing care, delayed respiratory depression should not be a problem. It is easily treated with naloxone. The delayed respiratory depression is always slow in onset—from the start of slowing of breathing it takes up to 45 min to reach a respiratory rate of less than 10 a minute, and longer than that for slower respiratory rates. Postoperative management then is simply a matter of recording the respiratory rate every 15 min to observe the trend. If the nursing staff are unable to do this they should not be looking after postoperative vascular surgery patients. This applies to the lesser varieties of vascular surgery, such as femoral–popliteal by-pass graft, carotid endarterectomy etc., where one can afford to be somewhat parsimonious with the dose of intrathecal morphine. Patients who have had more major vascular surgery should be in an intensive care unit where the standard of nursing should be higher. With this aggressive approach to postoperative pain it is possible to have a 75-year-old patient, 2 hours after having had an abdominal aortic aneurysm resected, sitting up in bed watching sport on television and cheering on his favourite team! The consequences, in terms of the reduction in postoperative pulmonary morbidity, are very substantial. The quality of the patients after intrathecal morphine is also slightly variable. Following all forms of vascular surgery covered with intrathecal morphine, approximately 20% of patients experience no pain at all throughout the whole postoperative period. The remainder experience some pain, which can vary from the relatively mild, which is controllable by simple oral non-narcotic analgesics, to moderately severe pain requiring powerful systemic opiate-type analgesics. If pain does occur, it is usually on the second or third postoperative day.

There are two disadvantages to the use of spinal morphine: one is the problem related to neostigmine that has been referred to earlier; the other is that when the analgesia wears off the patient becomes aware, for the first time, of what, for that operation, is the normal postoperative pain, if this should still be present. This can be very disturbing and requires specific educational effort if the patient is not to be unduly alarmed, as he is likely to attribute the emergence of severe pain, appearing perhaps days after operation, as signifying some new major postoperative complication. Equally, should the patient need further surgery at a later date and this is performed under a more conventional analgesic regimen, the experience of normal postoperative pain can be more than a little disconcerting, and evoke some very critical comment from the patient as he recalls his previous postoperative experiences.

Following the use of intrathecal morphine, a rare problem which can occur in the vascular surgery patient, is the development of acute opiate withdrawal symptoms (Messahel and Tomlin, 1981). Some patients, who have developed crescendo ischaemic rest pain prior to surgery, will have been receiving opiates for a variable period of time whilst their surgical problems were being evaluated. In this time the occasional patient can become addicted to the narcotic. Postoperatively, after receiving intrathecal morphine, such a patient can present a picture of obvious total analgesia, produced by the spinal morphine and yet have hallucinations, disorientation, mood changes, autonomic disturbances and all the other signs and symptoms characteristic of acute narcotic withdrawal. This problem arises because, although the spinal cord still has the morphine acting upon it, there is no morphine in the brain. This can be very disconcerting to the attending staff in that the patient is clearly responding to morphine yet apparently is not receiving morphine. Fortunately, this type of iatrogenic transient addiction is not long lasting and responds to conventional methods of treatment. This problem is novel in that had these patients been cared for by the customary use of postoperative systemic analgesics, they would not develop any withdrawal symptoms, as the gradual scaling down of their postoperative analgesics would have weaned them off their temporary addiction. Furthermore, because of conventional postoperative analgesic regimes, surgical staff would not anticipate acute narcotic withdrawal problems in the immediate postoperative period. It must be inferred that the same situation could occur in all patients who are addicted to narcotics.

Experience with other intrathecal narcotics in vascular surgery is somewhat limited but, characteristically, they have a shorter duration of action than morphine whilst conferring little additional benefit. However, this development is still in its early days and some of the newer analgesics, e.g. lofentanil or carfentanil or similiar derivatives may resolve the problem of profound, prolonged analgesia coupled with no respiratory depression. This, though, may be a philosopher's stone.

HAEMODYNAMIC CONSIDERATIONS

There are four possible combinations of blood pressure and flow that can be achieved, during anaesthesia, for patients undergoing surgery on the aorta or iliac vessels. Each can be achieved by a specific anaesthetic technique (*Table* 4.1).

Table 4.1

Circulation condition	Specimen anaesthetic technique
1. High pressure and high flow	N_2O + narcotic + relaxant
2. High flow and low pressure	Epidural block
3. Low flow and high pressure	Spinal plus vasoconstrictors
4. Low flow and low pressure	Deep halothane

The choice of anaesthetic technique is dictated by the circulatory conditions deemed best for the operation. The arguments for a low pressure system rest on the desire to achieve maximum peripheral vasodilatation so that all collateral vessels are opened in the area of surgery. Then, when the main stem artery is clamped off, the collateral vessels will maintain adequate flow and so prevent tissue hypoxia and the accumulation of acid metabolites. In fact, in patients with severe arterial disease, within the affected ischaemic zone all the collaterals that can be opened are open in response to the local tissue ischaemia and there is no reserve of blood vessels left to augment flow. This also explains the relative failure of sympathectomy in patients with ischaemic disease (Walker, 1982). Following epidural block, vessels within the zone of the block but outside the ischaemic zone are now dilated maximally so that the blood pressure falls. Outside the zone of the block, this fall in blood pressure will cause a marked fall in flow through any vessel whose lumen is partially blocked by rough patches of atheroma. This carries the risk of fresh thrombus formation and tissue infarction. A variation of this is that, distal to that patch of atheroma, the residual pressure, after the blood has squeezed through the narrowed vessel, may be below the critical opening pressure of the local arterioles. This is particularly applicable to the cerebral vessels and the mechanism is discussed more fully in Chapter 6 (p. 161) when considering anaesthesia for carotid artery surgery. Another hazard with this approach is the risk of clot formation in the actual vascular graft. Some grafts rely on platelet deposition in the interstices of the weave of the graft material for haemostasis. In turn, these grafts rely on the high-velocity bolus flow to sweep away any early fibrin/platelet aggregations that form on the side walls of the graft which would otherwise threaten to accumulate and eventually block the graft. These aggregations are subsequently broken up in the turbulent areas of blood flow, such as at arterial bifurcations distal to the graft. Any reduction of this scouring action increases the risk of graft failure. Low pressure and/or low flow systems therefore confer no benefit to the patient.

The epidural approach, usually performed under cover of a light general anaesthetic, has other problems. With an epidural block there is inhibition of vasoconstrictive fibres both at the arterioles and, more importantly, at the venuoles. As a result blood is sequestered in the small peripheral vessels. As a direct consequence the venous return falls, the cardiac output falls and the arterial pressure falls further. Such vessels that can vasoconstrict do so. These are the vessels outside the area covered by the epidural block. Thus, outside the area of the block, the flow is reduced, but within the zone of the block mass flow is increased although the velocity of flow in the individual smaller arteries is less. To counter the hypotension, it is prudent to give a vasoconstrictor agent. The effect of this sympathomimetic drug is principally at the arteriole. Systemic vascular resistance then increases, thus causing a rise in blood pressure. The venomotor tone also increases but to a lesser extent. The venous return increases but still does not return to normal. Cardiac output is still less than normal and the venous return needs to be augmented with an infusion of a crystalloid solution. Few vasoconstrictor drugs are pure adrenergic alpha-receptor stimulating agents, so inevitably there will be some adrenergic beta-receptor stimulation. This will increase myocardial contractility, but the key problem is still the venous return. The beta-receptor adrenergic stimulation may induce some cardiac ar-rhythmias particularly if the coronary circulation has some degree of partial atheromatous occlusion. Nevertheless, with the addition of the vasoconstrictor drug, the vasodilatation within the area of the epidural block is lessened, and mass flow falls. Any advantages of the high flow system are now largely gone. More important, the auto-regulatory system of control of blood pressure, regional flow and volume is now much less efficient. Against this pharmacological confusion, the ability to compensate for sudden haemorrhage and to redistribute the blood flow according to regional need, is seriously impaired.

Given that from the circulatory standpoint the epidural approach to anaesthesia for vascular surgery is not without its pitfalls, even if covered with a very light nitrous oxide and relaxant anaesthesia it is worth considering its advantages. There are two main advantages: (a) the quality of the analgesia is very high and (b) there is no need for centrally acting powerful drugs such as intravenous narcotics or inhalational vapours, which can disturb not only the vasomotor centre but also other centres such as the respiratory centre, the vomiting centre and the thermoregulatory centre.

Spinally applied opiates would seem to have all the advantages of the epidural approach with much fewer disadvantages. There is also very good and long lasting control of pain, and there is no disturbance of the circulatory system. The cardiovascular system can then respond very rapidly to changes in circulating blood volume.

Both the intravenous narcotic plus relaxant technique and the spinal narcotic plus relaxant technique produce a high-flow high-pressure situation and the whole circulation, in the elderly arteriopathic patient, behaves as a fixed pressure/volume system. These patients have poor powers of compensatory vasoconstriction which would otherwise sustain the blood pressure to near normal levels in the presence of a modest haemorrhage. Blood pressure, therefore, reflects circulating blood volume. There is one other aspect. Because of the loss of the diastolic pump effect due to a relatively inelastic aorta, these patients' hearts are working harder than normal. To sustain this effort requires a slightly raised left end-diastolic pressure. If the venous return falls the end-diastolic pressure falls (as the stroke volume falls ventricular emptying becomes more efficient). As the end-diastolic pressure falls so does myocardial contractility (Rusy, 1971). In these hard working hearts any small reduction in myocardial contractility leads to a precipitous fall in systolic blood pressure, although the diastolic pressure falls only slightly.

RHEOLOGICAL CONSIDERATIONS

There are two aspects of the rheology which need consideration: the first and more important is the maintenance of the circulating blood volume and the second is the question of inducing a mild degree of haemodilution. Inevitably, these two aspects are intertwined. During transfusion aimed at maintaining the circulating blood volume, particularly if the transfusion is a large one (over 3 l), the possibility of unintentionally inducing some degree of haemodilution should be borne in mind.

During vascular surgery the blood loss is unpredictable. However, it is important that the replacement fluid should keep up with the blood loss. Otherwise the arterial pressure falls, the cardiac output falls, coronary perfusion falls and myocardial contractility falls. It may take up to 15 min to recover from the hypotension even though the blood volume has been quickly restored to normal. The central venous pressure is a poor guide as to the adequacy of the circulating blood volume. Prevention of this hypotension is much more important than treating it.

During the surgery a variable portion of the vascular bed is clamped off. This may lead to a spuriously raised blood pressure as the circulating blood volume fills this restricted vascular bed. The true state of affairs may not be apparent until the vascular bed is returned to its normal size. It is prudent, therefore, to over-transfuse, by approximately 1-2 units of blood whilst the vascular bed is reduced. If the patient has severe ischaemic, or other major heart disease the patient's heart may not be able to cope adequately with this increased load. If this is the case, it is imperative to liaise with the surgeon, particularly at the time of releasing any arterial clamps. The clamp should be released very slowly with periods of partial occlusion whilst the blood pressure is constantly checked and further blood is given, titrating the volume infused against the blood pressure and, if possible, the central venous pressure. (In this particular circumstance, of a poorly functioning heart, the central venous pressure is a good guide as to the state of the right ventricle and the adequacy of the blood replacement.) Gradually the circulating blood volume is increased as the vascular bed is slowly enlarged. This approach is especially important when dealing with aortic aneurysms; it is less so in occlusive aorto-iliac disease as there will be already a number of collateral vessels taking blood from the upper trunk to the pelvis and beyond, so that the reduction of the vascular bed produced by the cross-clamp is less severe.

With surgery for a femoral–popliteal graft the problem is much less acute. Following a successful graft the average blood flow through such a graft, into one leg in an atherosclerotic patient, is of the order of 200–400 ml/min, i.e. less than 10% of the cardiac output of a lightly anaesthetized patient. Such an increase in demand of the cardiac output should be well within the capability of any patient likely to benefit from such an operation. There is one small caveat.

This relates to the in situ saphenous vein by-pass graft. In this operation the saphenous vein is left in place. Its side-branches are all tied off, the valves within the vein are surgically destroyed, the top and bottom ends of the vein are divided and the portion of vein in between is anastomosed to the femoral and tibial or peroneal arteries. Clearly if a major branch of the vein has not been tied off, much of the arterial blood, at the time of release of the arterial clamps, will flow through this—what is, essentially, an arterial venous fistula. The total blood flow through the graft can then be three or four times normal. A flow as much as 800–1000 ml/min is not impossible. This can make a very sizeable demand upon the cardiac output.

Haemoglobin solutions are very viscous and a solution of haemoglobin of 15 g per 100 ml of fluid has the viscosity of dilute treacle. Hence the haemoglobin is packed inside red cell envelopes which minimizes this viscosity yet has little effect upon gas transport and gaseous homeostasis. Nevertheless, at a haemoglobin concentration of 15 g% with all the red cells full of haemoglobin so that the mean corpuscular haemoglobin concentration (MCHC) is normal, this red-cell mass generates a haematocrit of 45%. Thus blood is not quite half full of semi-solids which are travelling as a homogeneous bolus all at the same velocity. This fluid still possesses a significant viscosity which requires work to push it through the orifices of the arterioles. Once beyond there, the axial streaming means that the viscous drag is that of plasma. Nevertheless, the work entailed in getting the blood through the arteriole is derived from the arterial blood pressure and so ultimately from the work done by the heart muscle.

If the haematocrit is reduced by diluting the blood with an appropriate fluid, this viscous drag is reduced. Thus for the same effort, or work, more flow would ensue, and this is augmented by vasodilatation. A delicate balance exists whereby the increased flow of the diluted blood compensates for the reduced oxygen content, per unit volume, of the blood, although this compensation is not quite complete (Daniel et al., 1986). Diluting the blood down to a haemoglobin concentration of 12 g% results in an unchanged or even improved oxygen supply to the tissues at a cost of increased flow or increased cardiac output, although the increase in cardiac work is proportionately less than the increase in cardiac output as the blood is less viscous. If the blood is diluted much lower than 12 g% the benefits of increased flow, due to the reduced viscosity, may be more than outweighed by the reduction in mass oxygen supply. A simple calculation shows that a 10% increase in flow combined with a 20% reduction in oxygen content results in a 12% reduction in mass oxygen supply; a 20% increase in flow with a 20% reduction in oxygen content results in a 4% reduction in total oxygen supply. It is not until the percentage increase in flow exceeds the percentage decrease in oxygen carrying capacity is there an increase in total oxygen supply. The objective, therefore, is for the increase in flow to exceed the effects of the haemodilution.

At the local level patches of atheroma create points of orificial flow—where flow is turbulent (and may be heard when listening over the vessel with a stethoscope). If turbulence is excessive, flow virtually ceases. Turbulence occurs when the Reynolds number is exceeded. The Reynolds number, in turn, depends upon the ratio of density to viscosity (Uvarov et al., 1973). Halving the viscosity without changing the density will double the Reynolds number. In fact, haemodilution techniques have very little effect on the density of blood; whole blood has a specific gravity of 1·06, whilst plasma has a specific gravity of 1·026 (Geigy, 1970). Thus, removing all the red cells results in a reduction in density of only approximately 3%. In contrast, whole blood has a viscosity of 2·5 centipoises (or mnewton-$\times$ sec/m^2) whereas for plasma the value is 1·1 centipoise. The viscosity of blood depends mainly on its red-cell content but the relationship between haematocrit and viscosity is not a linear one (Pirofsky, 1953). The addition of 1 l of saline to a blood volume of 5 l will reduce the haemoglobin by 17%, lower the haematocrit from 45% to 37·5%, reduce the dynamic viscosity by 19% and increase the Reynolds number by 24%. Since, within the circulation, the flow is close to the boundary between uniform flow and turbulent flow, e.g. it is uniform in the descending aorta but turbulent in the aortic arch (Tomlin and Duck, 1975), and at points of branching or narrowing, such an increase in the Reynolds number could well effect a marked increase in flow. If viscous drag through narrow atheromatous vessels, perhaps with turbulence, is the main impediment to blood flow and oxygen supply, then reducing the viscosity will lead to an increase in flow and oxygen supply. Clinically haemodilution has been found to be effective in patients with intermittent claudication (Yates et al., 1979). Saline, though, is not an appropriate haemodiluent as it leaves the circulation too quickly. Low molecular weight dextrans would have a similar effect but would remain in the circulation. Plasma would not be so efficient as the plasma proteins would, in their own right, make a small but significant contribution to the viscosity. Haemodilution techniques also come into their own when the haematocrit is abnormally high, as the viscosity rises increasingly sharply the higher the haematocrit (Pirofsky, 1953). One particular effect of haemodilution is to increase cerebral blood flow. This is because cerebral blood flow is determined to a large extent by the oxygen content of the arterial blood (Brown et al., 1985). If the oxygen content is inadequate local metabolites accumulate and cause vasodilatation.

When considering patients with arterial disease who have undergone surgery, the potential benefits of haemodilution become magnified. The surgical wound evokes an inflammatory response. Part of that response is a localized hyperaemia, as many capillaries open up to provide the inflammatory exudate, fibrin formation and eventually the scaffold for the healing tissue. In normal subjects there is no problem in increasing the blood supply to meet this augmented demand. More capillaries open up, the arterial flow increases and the viscosity of the blood is of little significance. In the arteriopathic patient this may not be the situation. The ability to increase flow may be limited because of partial occlusion of the major feeding vessels. Hence, if flow can be facilitated by reducing the viscosity of the blood more oxygen can be supplied to the healing wound. There is, therefore, a reasonable argument for haemodiluting the patients during the anaesthesia for vascular surgery. The timing of the haemodilution is important and there must be no contra-indications —of which the principal one is ischaemic heart disease.

Patients with ischaemic heart disease are already extracting maximally the oxygen in the arterial blood of the coronary vasculature. The end-capillary oxygen tension, particularly of the subendocardial vessels is very, very low, and may be approaching an oxygen tension of less than $0 \cdot 1$ kPa (less than 10 mmHg). If the blood is haemodiluted, the increased coronary flow may not carry enough oxygen to meet the normal metabolic demand, let alone any augmented demand resulting from an increase in cardiac output consequent upon the iatrogenically induced anaemia. Flow in the subendocardial vessels is dictated not only by the arterial blood pressure and the viscosity of the blood but also, and more importantly, by the duration of diastole (Guyton, 1981). Any tachycardia resulting from the increase in cardiac output, consequent upon the haemodilution, may erode that diastolic time. (The initial response to haemodilution is an increase in sympathetic drive to increase the cardiac output. This generates a mild tachycardia. This, in turn, shortens both systole and diastole, but in mild tachycardia the systolic time is shortened more than the diastolic time so that, per minute, more time is spent in diastole (Ganong, 1983). As the tachycardia increases, to over 100 beats per minute, the shortening of systole gradually reaches a maximum and any further increase in heart rate is achieved by shortening the diastolic time. This means that, as the tachycardia increases, less time is available, per minute, for perfusing the subendocardial vessels.) Further, the increase in cardiac output consequent upon the iatrogenic anaemia or haemodilution requires some increased work from the heart. This in turn increases the output flow, velocity, energy requirements and oxygen demand by the cardiac muscle. But the reduction, if not loss, of the diastolic pump effect, normally produced by an elastic aorta, means that greater work is thrown on the left ventricle. The end result is that, if there is marked ischaemic heart disease and a severe loss of aortic elasticity, anything more than a very mild haemodilution will cause a reduction in myocardial oxygenation at a time when the heart is being asked to work harder.

The other aspect of haemodilution that needs some consideration is that the circulating blood volume should be normal. Otherwise, there is a smaller volume of blood to be diluted and if normal volumes of diluent are given the end result will be an excessive haemodilution.

The timing of the haemodilution is important. If it is done early in surgery and there is marked blood loss, then some of the blood loss will be of haemodiluted blood. The excess loss will be or should be replaced by whole blood and, therefore, at the end of operation the much-sought-after improvement in blood viscosity consequent upon the haemodilution will be lost. It follows that haemodilution is best performed near the end of operation, after the various phases of maximum likelihood of major haemorrhage. The simplest way is to replace with the diluent the oozing that occurs through the graft after the graft has been opened up to the circulation.

Blood has a high oxygen-carrying capacity but transfused blood is qualitatively different from normal blood. It is diluted with a citrate solution and has no calcium ions. Its haemoglobin concentration and haematocrit are somewhat lower than normal. As a vehicle for delivering oxygen to the tissues, transfused blood is less efficient than normal blood and this reduction in oxygen transport efficiency increases with the duration of extracorporeal storage of the blood. This reduction in the efficiency of haemoglobin in releasing oxygen at low oxygen tension levels is due to a loss of 2,3-diphosphoglycerate (DPG) (Valtis and Kennedy, 1954; Akerblom et al., 1968). Notwithstanding this, total exchange transfusions are not uncommon during aortic aneurysm surgery, especially if the aneurysm is ruptured, and the oxygen-carrying capacity of the transfused blood is more than adequate for survival. This effect has also been confirmed experimentally (Collins, 1980). Even so, where very large blood transfusions are necessary, it is important to increase the arterial oxygen tension well above normal in order to increase the arterial-peripheral tissue oxygen tension gradient. The mass transfer of oxgyen to the peripheral tissues is thus aided. It is in this area that the deficiencies in oxygen transport have their effect. The oxygen transfer defect is not long lasting; 25% of the 2,3-DPG is restored within 3 hours, and 50% within 5–24 hours (Valleri and Hirsh, 1969).

Following blood transfusion, the citrate is metabolized and metabolized very quickly. At normothermia, the metabolism of citrate is such that the total citrate in 2 units of blood is cleared within 1 min. This is not true if hypothermia has developed to any significant extent (below 35 °C—a situation not uncommon during aortic surgery). At faster rates of blood transfusion, beyond 2 units/min, then the citrate will need neutralizing, and the ionized calcium will need elevating, otherwise there will be marked myocardial depression and a severe reduction in myocardial contractility. It is a good, if somewhat empirical, practice to give 2·5 mmol of calcium ions for every 1–2 units of blood after the first 3 units of blood. In this way undue lowering of the ionized serum calcium concentration will be avoided.

When the citrate is metabolized, the water in which the citrate was dissolved escapes into the extracellular fluid and the intracellular space. The osmolality of the blood therefore changes very little. A similar situation occurs with crystalloid solutions. Diluting the blood with crystalloid solution merely increases the volume of the extracellular fluid. This is relevant when considering the use of blood concentrates or packed cells in which the plasma, with all its clotting factors and serum proteins, has been removed, or 'harvested'. The ratio of interstitial fluid to intravascular fluid is about 3 : 1 (Keele et al., 1982). It requires four times as much crystalloid solution to restore the functional volume of a unit of red-cell concentrate to normal as it does plasma. Giving the packed cells, or blood concentrate, undiluted has two disadvantages. The first is purely technical. It is very difficult to give at a high flow rate but high flow rates of the transfused blood are not infrequently required during vascular surgery. The second disadvantage is that it is very viscous and so will raise the blood viscosity which will reduce blood flow in zones of ischaemia. The concentrate must be diluted. Diluting the blood with plasma or a colloid solution reduces the viscosity of the blood and this improves the perfusion of the micro-circulation and, therefore, improves the delivery of oxygen to the tissues and so the oxygen uptake and utilization. Nevertheless, the total supply of oxygen is, in the absence of hypoxia, more than enough to cope with this increased utilization.

The extent of how far one can proceed with this haemodilution is a matter of debate. It would seem logical to replace the volume of anticoagulant solution in transfused blood with fresh frozen plasma, as this volume of anticoagulant will be lost from the circulation, and then to ignore this volume of plasma in the calculation of the blood balance. Since the volume of anticoagulant in a unit of blood is approximately 20% of the total, this means giving 1 unit of fresh frozen plasma for every 5 units of blood. Fresh frozen plasma has some marginal advantages over synthetic colloids or even purified protein fraction (PPF), in that it does contain useful quantities of various clotting factors and it does not interfere with blood cross-matching, should any additional cross-matching of blood become necessary. Fresh frozen or reconstituted freeze-dried plasma does have a small but definite risk of carrying the hepatitis B virus. This risk is very difficult to quantitate as the incidence of infective hepatitis varies over a 4–5 year cycle against a steadily rising background. (At least, this is the situation in the United Kingdom; in other countries the epidemiology of hepatitis is very different.) Hence, the degree of contamination will depend upon whether there was a minor epidemic at the time of blood donation with the possibility of some of the donors either incubating or suffering from a sub-clinical attack of hepatitis. The risk of hepatitis increases in those countries where the disease is endemic. A more recent anxiety is the question of the blood or plasma carrying the virus responsible for AIDS (Acquired Immune Deficiency Syndrome). For emergency circulatory support the use of plasma has largely been replaced by the use of gelatins.

Apart from the haemodilution that accompanies blood tranfusion there are several other ways of producing the desired reduction in blood viscosity. These are to give a diluent and the choice lies between:

1. The dextrans
2. The albumin solutions
3. The gelatins
4. The crystalloid solutions
5. The hydroxy-ethyl starch
6. The fluorocarbons

1. The dextrans

There are two commonly used dextrans, Dextran 40 and Dextran 70. Dextran 40 has a molecular weight averaging around 40 000 daltons. It is slightly hyperosmolar and will expand the blood volume in part by its own volume and in part by drawing water from the interstitial space—the ratio being very nearly 50 : 50. Dextran 70 has a higher average molecular weight and hence the number of osmotically active ingredients is less. It has, therefore, a less dehydrating effect on the interstitial space. The kidneys can excrete up to 5 g of dextran per day so the dextrans may stay in the circulation for a number of days but this depends upon the size of the molecule of dextran. Fifty per cent of Dextran 40 will be excreted by the kidney within 3 hours, as compared with 30% of Dextran 70 in 6 hours, and 40% of the rarely used Dextran 110 in 24 hours (Pharmaceutical Codex, 1979b). If more than 1·5 l of dextran are given at any one time this can induce significant disturbances of the blood so that cross-matching may be seriously perturbed. This, too, is a function of molecular size, the larger the molecule the greater the disturbance.

2. The albumin solutions

These are available in several forms. The commonest is purified protein fraction (PPF). Essentially, this is a simple blood extract from which all the red cells, clotting factors and larger proteins have been removed. It consists of an almost pure 5% albumin solution. Higher concentrations of albumin, up to a 20% concentration, are also commercially available. Albumin is readily metabolized by the liver —particularly in the metabolically depleted patient, and it rarely stays in the circulation for more than 24–48 hours (Schultze and Heremans, 1966). It has, therefore, limited value as a haemodiluting agent. The osmotic pressure of PPF is the same as whole blood, but the 20% solution is hyperosmolar and so will cause some reduction in the size of the extra-vascular compartments, most notably of the intracellular compartment. The albumin solutions carry a small but definite risk of generating an allergic reaction, and they also contain some bradykinin. Nevertheless, as temporary support of the circulation the albumin solutions are better than the dextrans.

3. The gelatins

These have a wide range of molecular weight from 5000 to 50 000 daltons. As a result, when given intravenously, some of the gelatin will leak out of the circulation into the extracellular fluid and some will leak out through the renal glomeruli. This will provoke a mild osmotic diuresis. The half-life of the gelatins is only 2–3 hours (Ring et al., 1980), which is insignificant when considering haemodilution as a potential aid to postoperative healing in the arteriopathic subject. The main value of the gelatins is for transient circulatory support during acute blood loss whilst awaiting cross-matched blood, e.g. during the management of a ruptured aortic aneurysm. The gelatins do contain significant amounts of ionized calcium and so should not be used in infusion lines that are used for the giving of whole blood. Allergic reactions are commoner after gelatin infusions than with any other plasma substitute (Mollison, 1983).

4. The crystalloid solutions

Simple crystalloid solutions will also act as haemodiluting agents, but they readily pass into the extracellular fluid. Since the ratio of extracellular to intravascular fluid volume is approximately 3 : 1 the crystalloid solutions will be split into this ratio, so that only one-quarter of the crystalloid will remain in the circulation. This split is achieved within 5–15 minutes of intravenous administration. Given normal postoperative kidney function the excess crystalloid will be excreted by the kidneys within 12–24 hours, and hence the benefit of haemodilution will be lost by then. In a recent review a persuasive case has been made out for a reduction in the use of crystalloids and a greater use of colloids during anaesthesia and surgery (Twigley and Hillman, 1985).

Dextrose solutions have no place in haemodilution. The sugar content is rapidly metabolized and the residual water will be distributed between all the water compartments in proportion to their relative size. This means that about 7% of the dextrose solution will remain within the circulation for haemodilution purposes. Even this will be excreted by the kidney within a few hours. Although the sugar content is rapidly metabolized, this takes place mainly after the anaesthetic as, during anaesthesia, the patient behaves like a diabetic and cannot metabolize sugar so readily (Allison et al., 1969).

5. Hydroxyethyl starch (HES)

Hydroxyethyl starch has been suggested by Rudowski and Kostra-zewska (1976). The particulate matter of hydroxyethyl starch has a molecular weight of 450 000 daltons and it is available as a 6% solution in normal saline. It does stay well in the body with a half-life of about 17 days. Potentially, it is a very useful haemodiluting agent but clinical experience with this agent is very limited. Only time will tell.

6. The fluorocarbons

Considerable interest has been shown in the use of the fluorocarbons (Jones, 1983). These are a family of simple organic molecules in which all the hydrogen atoms have been replaced by fluorine. Chemically they are very inert and yet they have a high capacity for carrying oxygen and carbon dioxide (Geyer, 1982). There is a curvilinear relationship between the oxygen-carrying capacity and the volatility or boiling point of the different fluorocarbons. Thus perfluoropentane, C_5F_{10} (boiling point 29 °C), when exposed to 100% oxygen, can carry 54 ml O_2/100 g, the equivalent figure for C_6F_{12} (boiling point 57 °C) is 41 ml O_2/100 g and for $C_{10}F_{22}$ (B.P. 142 °C) 24·4 ml O_2/100 g. Fluorocarbons have a high specific gravity, of between 1·75 and 2·0. Since fluorocarbons can be more or less tailor manufactured to different boiling points this means that the ideal fluorocarbon with a boiling point of 45 °C (any lower boiling point would risk intravascular vaporization, with the catastrophic production of multiple gas emboli) would have an oxygen-carrying capacity of 45 ml O_2/100 g. Such a compound, at a fluorocrit of 50% when exposed to an arterial oxygen tension of 14 kPa, would be able to carry about 6 ml O_2%, c.f. 20 ml O_2% for whole blood at Hb 15 g%. The respective figures when exposed to an oxygen tension of 5·6 kPa are 2·5 ml O_2% as compared with 15 ml O_2% for venous blood. Thus the best that can be hoped for when breathing air with a 50% v/v concentration of perfluorocarbon (so leaving space for the plasma proteins, etc.) is only as good as blood with an Hb level of 11–12 g%. Furthermore, should the tissue oxygen tension fall with the perfluorocarbons there is little reserve of additional oxygen available as compared with whole blood. However, in the case of the fluorocarbons, the tissue oxygen supply can be very significantly increased by augmenting the inspired oxygen concentration. Raising the arterial oxygen tension to around 28 kPa (by increasing the inspired oxygen concentration to 35–40%) will almost quadruple the tissue oxygen supply with such a fluorocarbon at this fluorocrit, as compared with only a marginal increase in tissue oxygen availability when dealing with whole blood. The main difficulty with the fluorocarbons is that they are extremely insoluble and so have to be emulsified. They are also very poor solvents so that the choice of emulsifying agents is limited, and this is particularly so for the smaller, lower molecular weight fluorocarbons. As an oxygen-carrying haemodiluent some limited clinical experience, using a 20% emulsion of fluorocarbon has been obtained (Mitsuno et al., 1982) in improving tissue oxygenation in severely ischaemic organs, but the incidence of adverse reactions to the emulsifying agents was high (Geyer, 1982; Long, 1982). Work on these compounds has been confined mainly to animals. At the moment they are more a tribute to the chemist's ingenuity than of much clinical value for everyday anaesthesia.

CLINICAL MANAGEMENT

Whilst the general principles of clinical anaesthesia for vascular surgery are much the same as for any major abdominal operation yet there are a few specific points which need emphasizing when giving an anaesthetic to a patient undergoing major vascular surgery. What follows represents the distillation of the author's experience of over 20 years as a vascular anaesthetist.

Premedication

This is discussed more fully in Chapter 2. Elderly patients presenting for vascular surgery rarely need any premedication.

Induction

The choice of induction agent is wide and will depend upon the anaesthetist's preference, subject to any pharmacological idiosyncrasies or sensitivities. The arteriopathic patient commonly has a very slow vein–artery, and so vein–brain, circulation time. Tests, using indocyanine green as a marker during cardiac output studies, have shown that it can take up to 90 s for the dye injected into a vein in the antecubital fossa to appear at the opposite radial artery. In contrast, the normal time in the young healthy subject is usually less than 30 s. This very slow circulating time can be a trap for the unwary and may lead to an unintentional overdose of the induction agent.

Recent work (Milocco et al., 1985) has shown that following induction of anaesthesia, irrespective of induction agent, the arteriopathic patient suffers a sharp reduction of left ventricular function, although this does respond to external stimuli unless the patient is very deeply narcotized.

Intubation

The technique for intubation will also depend upon the anaesthetist's preference. Given the slow circulating time, intubation using a non-depolarizing long-acting muscle relaxant can lead to a very protracted intubation with the risk of the induction agent wearing off before the intubation has been completed. Given the average duration of operating time for most vascular surgery, there seems no significant contra-indication to the use of succinylcholine for intubation. Problems related to dual block, scoline apnoea and the like will all have worn off before the operation is completed. Since these arteriopathic patients withstand hypoxia so badly, it seems reasonable to have the optimum intubation conditions and institute artificial ventilation as soon as possible.

Following the induction of anaesthesia, the various lines and cannulas that will be used for monitoring or transfusion are established. If the patient has large veins, then a single blood transfusion line is all that is necessary. If the proposed operation is on the aorta or iliac arteries and the veins are not particularly large, then two transfusion lines should be established (unless there is a central venous pressure line set up). Since during the operation the surgeon will be standing on the patient's right side, it is useful to insert the lines, including the arterial line, in the left arm and have this abducted and lying on a board at right-angles to the patient's body. The anaesthetist will then have easy access to the veins for drug administration. More importantly, he will be able to see the entire length of the lines and detect and correct any inadvertent disconnection or kinking. This can happen at any time, but particularly during periods of very rapid blood transfusion under pressure and when the connections are simple push-fit ones. Luer-Lok connections should be used wherever possible. If the lines are covered by the surgical drapes, this poses an unnecessary if remote hazard. In thoracic vascular or carotid artery surgery it may not be feasible to have the arm abducted, in which case especial care should be taken as to the security of the various drip connections.

Maintenance

The triad of (1) sleep, (2) relaxation and (3) analgesia applies to the vascular patient just as much as they apply to the general surgical patient.

1. Sleep

Sleep is best maintained with nitrous oxide. However, the concentration of nitrous oxide unless intrathecal narcotics are being used should not exceed 65%, except when facilities are available for blood-gas measurements during anaesthesia. These patients are already hypoxaemic as a result of the ageing process. In addition, they develop, during anaesthesia, marked intrapulmonary shunting with significant disturbances of the ventilation/perfusion ratio (VA/Q) such that to maintain the arterial oxygen tension to near normal levels in these patients commonly requires an inspired oxygen concentration of 35% or more (De Almeida, 1975). If intrathecal narcotics are used, the inspired oxygen concentration can be lowered to 25% and the nitrous oxide concentration raised to 75% and yet the same arterial oxygen tensions will result. Why this is so remains a mystery. If blood-gas measurement facilities are available during the operation, the concentration of inspired nitrous oxide may be titrated against the arterial oxygen tension so that the inspired nitrous oxide concentration is raised without producing hypoxaemia.

In a proportion of patients this 65% concentration of nitrous oxide may not be enough to subdue all awareness and a supplemental agent may be necessary. If intravenous narcotics are being used, particularly if either fentanyl or phenoperidine coupled with droperidol are being used, this will provide sufficient additional sedation for it to be extremely unlikely that the patient will develop any awareness. Intravenous morphine is not so good in this respect. The alternative is a trace of inhalational vapour. If an intrathecal narcotic has been used, the need for inhalational supplement is increased, despite the ability to use a slightly higher concentration of nitrous oxide without producing hypoxaemia.

Apart from nitrous oxide, inhalational agents do present some problems. Volatile anaesthetic agents, even with nitrous oxide, should not be used to the level where they produce surgical muscle relaxation. The degree of depression of the vasomotor system that results when this depth of anaesthesia is reached can be life-threatening in the patient with widespread arterial disease. Anaesthetic vapours can, however, be used in much lower concentrations as an adjuvant when muscle relaxants are used. Even then there are difficulties.

Halothane is contra-indicated in major vascular surgery, especially if the patient is hypertensive (as the majority are). In the hypertensive arteriopathic patient the heart has had to hypertrophy to maintain a normal cardiac output. It is working much harder than in the normal patient. As a consequence, the heart is particularly sensitive to any agent that has myocardial depressant properties. (It is axiomatic in anaesthesia that any physiological system or organ which is working harder than usual is unduly sensitive to any depressant effect produced by any anaesthetic drugs. Examples are legion: the respiratory system in airways obstruction from laryngeal cancer, the asthmatic, the myasthenic, the blood-volume-depleted trauma patient and so on.) Halothane, even in concentrations as low as 0·5%, can cause marked hypotension and, more importantly, a very sluggish vascular system that responds slowly and poorly to sudden changes in haemodynamics—whether due to the surgeon unexpectedly losing rapidly a large volume (more than 200 ml in 10 s) of blood or rapidly altering the size of the vascular bed.

Isoflurane has proved to be disappointing when used in arterial surgery. In concentrations as low as 0·5% (*Fig.* 4.4) it can produce marked hypotension. The physical characteristics of isoflurane enable it to be cleared from the body very quickly, so that correction of the sluggishness of the reactivity of the vascular system is much less of a problem than it is with halothane. Whilst its minimal disturbance of the heart's conducting system may be considered by some as an advantage, yet its hypotensive properties are a major drawback to its use in anaesthesia for vascular surgery.

Enflurane in concentrations of between 0·25% and 0·5% provides a sufficient increase in depth of anaesthesia to prevent any awareness and yet produces minimal disturbances of the circulatory system. Even in concentrations as high as 1–2% in severely hypertensive patients the disturbances of blood pressure are slow, gradual in onset and easy and quick to reverse (*Fig.* 4.5). It is thus the inhalational agent of choice as a supplementary drug to nitrous oxide for the patient requiring anaesthesia for vascular surgery. Attempts have been made to rely solely on enflurane to provide sleep during vascular surgery (with analgesia controlled by intrathecal morphine and muscle relaxation by the use of muscle relaxants), the enflurane being vaporized in a mixture of oxygen and air. Since nitrous oxide reduces

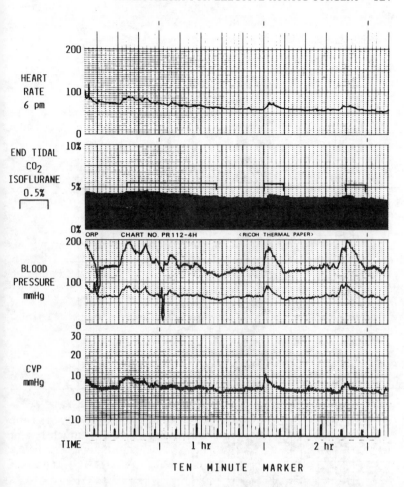

Fig. 4.4.   **The effects of isoflurane on blood pressure during arterial surgery. A typical record, this is from a male, aged 70, undergoing femoral
popliteal by-pass surgery. Anaesthesia: methohexitone, nitrous oxide, pancuronium, intrathecal morphine, and intermittent isoflurane 0·5 %. The
isoflurane produced a progressive fall in systolic blood pressure of
50–70 mmHg to 110–120 mmHg, then following discontinuing the isoflurane
the blood pressure remained stable for more than 20 min. When recovery did
occur it was very sudden and was associated with a sharp rise in blood
pressure as well as small increases in heart rate, central venous pressure and
in end-tidal CO_2 concentration—all due to a peripheral vasoconstrictive
effect leading to an increase in venous return and cardiac output and so blood
pressure. As can be seen, these effects were repeatable in this patient. (Heart
rate in beats per minute.)**
(Previously unpublished data.)

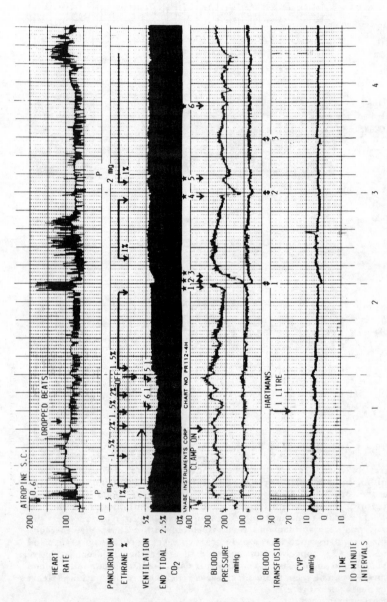

```
*1  Clamp release Rt.leg      *4 = Clamp release Lt.leg
*2  Clamp On                  *5 = Clamp On
*3  Clamp release Slowly      *6 · Fem-Pop Lt leg Clamp Release
```

Fig. 4.5.   The effects of arterial clamp release. A complete record of a 72-year-old male, severely hypertensive (resting blood pressure 270/150 mmHg), undergoing aorto-bifemoral graft and a femoral popliteal by-pass graft for pregangrene.

Upper trace: Heart rate (beats per minute). This shows the effect of subcutaneous atropine 0·6 mg After it had worn off, at 45 min, the patient developed occasional ectopic beats which could drop the heart rate. Spikes on record are diathermy artefacts.

Second trace: End-tidal CO_2 and enflurane concentration. Note the progressive reduction in minute volume from 7 to 5 l/min in order to maintain the same end tidal CO_2 .Note also that within 3 min of discontinuing the enflurane (at time 2 hours 5 min) the blood pressure rose from 200 to 280 mmHg. There was a similar but slower response near the end of the anaesthetic.

Third trace: Blood pressure. The enflurane appeared to block any hypertensive response when the aortic clamp was applied. When the clamp was released to the right leg the systolic pressure fell precipitously from 275 to 100 mmHg. Within 2 min the clamp was reapplied and when the blood pressure regained 200 mmHg it was released slowly over 2 min. Meanwhile a blood transfusion was started.

Bottom trace: Central venous pressure. The hypotension was accompanied by a small but sharp fall in central venous pressure. A similar episode occurred when the clamp was released to the left leg. The clamp was reapplied for further aterial surgery to the leg and when the clamp was released (at 3 hours 50 min) there was no hypotension—as the circulating blood volume had been expanded by blood transfusion to create a small rise of 2 mmHg in central venous pressure.

(Previously unpublished data.)

the MAC (or minimum alveolar concentration for anaesthesia) value of enflurane, the concentration of administered vapour needs to be increased. This, in turn, increases the risk of hypotension during anaesthesia. There is one practical disadvantage in this type of approach. The anaesthetist is crucially dependent upon the correct and efficient operation of the vaporizer, otherwise awareness (in a paralysed patient) or over-dosage may result. In contrast when nitrous oxide is being used, the anaesthetist can see the rotameter bobbin moving and so will have greater confidence that, all other things being equal, the patient is receiving what the anaesthetist desires him to receive.

2. Relaxation

Muscle relaxation may be achieved with any of the non-depolarizing relaxants. Tubocurarine is relatively contra-indicated as it possesses weak ganglion-blocking properties (Taylor, 1980) and so can induce a mild hypotension. More importantly, during tubocurarine relaxation the circulatory system is somewhat sluggish to adjust to any abrupt changes in circulatory haemodynamics. Pancuronium produces profound relaxation, but the question has been raised, and not yet answered, that the postoperative hypertension which occurs after any major vascular operation is greater in those patients who have been given pancuronium than in those patients who have received alcuronium or any other non-depolarizing relaxant. Apart from tubocurarine, there is very little to choose between these various relaxants and so the choice will depend upon the anaesthetist's familiarity with the drugs and his personal preference.

Following the relaxant, the patient must be artificially ventilated. Vascular patients present no undue problems as far as this is concerned, unless there is associated obstructive airways disease present when the normal precautions and methods of management apply. Artificial ventilation is best adjusted to maintain the Pa_{CO_2} slightly below normal, an end-tidal CO_2 monitor is invaluable here, as during the operation the patient is likely to develop a degree of hypothermia. This will both lower his metabolic rate and his carbon dioxide output markedly. An end-tidal CO_2 monitor will enable the anaesthetist to maintain the end-expired carbon dioxide concentration to between 4 and 5%. This will ensure that there is no excessive over-ventilation which could adversely affect the venous return.

If the ventilator available has the facility to supply a falling flow pattern of ventilation, this will give the best arterial oxygen tension for any given inspired oxygen concentration, although the gains achieved over the more common constant flow ventilators are somewhat less than 1 kPa (De Almeida, 1975). Slow deep inspirations, with an inspiratory–expiratory ratio of 1 : 3 and at a frequency of about 10 breaths per minute, appear to provide the optimum haemodynamics, particularly if the tidal volume is adjusted to maintain the end-expired carbon dioxide concentration to between 4 and 5%. With this arrangement and with no rebreathing, minute volumes of about 6 l/min are normal, dropping to 4·5–5 l/min as the operation progresses. In the older patients (80+ years) these volumes can be reduced by 15–25%. If an end-tidal carbon dioxide monitor is not available, then artificial ventilation should err on the high side, balancing the ventilation against the central venous pressure and blood pressure. This is preferable as under-ventilation carries with it the risk of carbon dioxide retention with its associated risk of arrhythmias. Patients with occlusive coronary disease have a lower Pa_{CO_2} arrhythmic threshold with hypercapnia as compared with other patients, and it is a wise precaution to assume that all older patients presenting for vascular surgery, potentially, have some degree of occlusive coronary artery disease.

3. Analgesia

When considering analgesia it is necessary to take into account not only intra-operative analgesia but also postoperative analgesia. The choice of analgesic regimen lies between intravenous narcotics and either epidural or intrathecal narcotics. The intravenous approach also lies between either periodic bolus doses of the narcotic of one's choice or narcotic by constant infusion pump (Catling et al., 1980; Rutter et al., 1980). The best studied of the latter is morphine by constant infusion. A number of similar methods with minor variations have been devised but one of the simplest techniques is to give a loading dose of 5–10 mg of morphine intravenously at the start of the anaesthetic followed by infusion of morphine at a rate of 1–2 mg/h. This can be maintained more or less indefinitely into the postoperative period with the rate of morphine infusion adjusted to between 1 and 4 mg/h dependent upon the patient's fluctuating needs. Postoperative pain is highly variable with time, being cyclic and reaching its first maximum at about 6 hours after anaesthesia (Gjessing and Tomlin, 1979), and thereafter waxing and waning in progressively longer cycles of lowered amplitude until severe pain is no longer felt. This can take up to 5 days if the patient has had an aortic aneurysmectomy, but is less after a femoral–popliteal by-pass operation. Inevitably with the constant infusion system the patient will feel some pain at some time, and the quality of the analgesia will depend upon the vigilance of the nursing and other attending staff in detecting the need to increase the rate of morphine infusion. Even then, given the slow onset time of morphine analgesia, the patient will feel some pain at the peak of the pain cycles, notwithstanding the staff being very prompt at adjusting the rate of morphine infusion as and when required. Nevertheless, the quality of the analgesia produced is a marked improvement over the alternative of predetermined doses of narcotic given on a fixed-time basis, although it does not give the more uniform spread of analgesia that can be achieved with intrathecal morphine.

The alternative, which is the author's preference, is to use intrathecal morphine, the rationale of which has been discussed earlier in this chapter (p. 108).

Anaesthesia reversal

There are no specific contra-indications to the use of neostigmine, preceded by atropine, to reverse the muscle relaxant in the vascular surgical patient. As has been discussed elsewhere (p. 100), if intrathecal narcotics have been used the neostigmine may cause some temporary colic, unless the patient has been pretreated with subcutaneous atropine at least 1 hour earlier. If colic should occur, it will respond to intravenous pethidine, and this, in turn, will wear off long before any of the intrathecal narcotic reaches the brain stem. If the operation has lasted more than 2–3 hours and the intrathecal morphine was given just after the induction of anaesthesia, the patient is highly unlikely to feel any colic.

Inevitably, at the end of operation these patients will have a somewhat lowered cardiac output if only because of their attendant hypothermia. Patients with a low cardiac output have a more intense degree of postoperative diffusion hypoxia (Scrimshire and Tomlin, 1973). These patients already have some degree of hypoxaemia, in part due to their own ageing process and in part due to the effects of the operation. To this is now added the accentuated diffusion hypoxia. At the end of operation, if severe hypoxaemia is to be avoided, these patients should be given a heavily enriched oxygen–air mixture to breathe, for approximately 5 min, to tide them over the diffusion hypoxia stage.

Thereafter, the arterial oxygen tension will improve over the next 2 hours, although it still will not reach its preoperative value, when it will decline to reach its nadir at about 6 hours after surgery (corresponding in time to the peak of the pain cycle). The postoperative hypoxaemia will then slowly improve but will not reach normal levels (after allowing for the age effect) for several days. This presumably again is due to subliminal pain, as the intensity of the postoperative hypoxaemia is reduced by half in those patients who have received intrathecal morphine, and this occurs even in those patients who appear to have perfect analgesia. Why there is this association between hypoxaemia and pain is not known. It is prudent, therefore, to give all arterial surgery patients additional oxygen to breathe for a prolonged period postoperatively.

KEY STAGES

During aortic surgery there are a number of stages during the anaesthetic and operation where untoward events are more likely to happen. Some are common to all major abdominal operations, others are specific to this type of surgery.

Induction

Following induction of anaesthesia, there may be a marked but transient hypotension, which may well last longer than the pharmacological duration of action of the induction agent. The vasomotor centre would appear to have lost its normal reactivity. The situation is analogous to the behaviour of the respiratory centre at the end of a prolonged nitrous oxide, artificial ventilation anaesthetic, when the respiratory centre needs a sudden stimulus to make it resume normal activity. The hypotension responds only slowly to a rapid infusion of a large volume (5–700 ml) of crystalloids, although the infusion will prevent the hypotension from deepening. In contrast, the skin incision or any sudden sharp cutaneous stimulus will provoke a very brisk return of the blood pressure to normal levels. Thereafter, the reactivity of the vasomotor centre remains normal.

Posterior peritoneal traction

During his surgical approach to the aorta, the surgeon must reflect the mesentery and posterior peritoneum for access to the aorta. This is, potentially, a particularly painful procedure and, if the analgesia is inadequate, there will be a pronounced autonomic response—commonly of bradycardia and hypotension. Although this will respond to intravenous atropine, yet the underlying cause—pain—must also be treated.

Aortic cross-clamping

This usually provokes a marked rise in systemic blood pressure as the heart is faced suddenly with a substantial increase in aortic impedance and a reduced vascular bed. This problem is greatest in those patients with an aortic aneurysm and who have a good run-off of flow to the lower limbs. It is less of a problem in those patients with occlusive aorto-iliac disease, who have had time to develop many collateral vessels to maintain a blood supply to the lower limbs and pelvis. The problem is normally self-limiting as the vasomotor centre and the heart adjust to the changes in haemodynamics. However, if the hypertension is very severe, it can be overcome by allowing fluid or blood replacement to fall behind blood loss. If the cross-clamp is applied at the level of the diaphragm, for suprarenal vascular surgery, it may be necessary to use a rapidly acting and short-acting vaso-dilator, such as sodium nitroprusside, in order to avoid acute left ventricular strain and left-sided heart failure. Before the aortic cross-clamp is released, it will be necessary to get back into positive blood balance ready for the re-expansion of the vascular bed.

Aortic clamp release

This is the most testing time during the whole anaesthetic period. During the period of cross-clamping some of the blood in the venous side of the circulation from the legs will have returned to the central circulation, propelled there by the venomotor tone. This blood in the legs will not have been replaced. The legs have a normal capacity of approximately half a litre of blood, but this capacity will have been augmented by the increased demand for flow consequent upon the local anoxia and metabolic acidosis which has occurred within the legs during the period of circulatory occlusion. In addition, when the flow is re-established there may be leaks of blood from the anastomotic sites or from the interstices of the graft material. Ideally, the circulating blood volume should have been augmented prior to aortic clamp release to the level where the central venous pressure rises one or two centimetres of water pressure above normal. If, on releasing the aortic cross-clamp, the blood pressure falls too sharply, the surgeon should be asked to reapply the clamp (*Fig.* 4.5), whilst more blood is rapidly transfused. When the blood pressure has returned to normal, the surgeon is asked to release the clamp more slowly, balancing the rate of release of the clamp against the arterial blood pressure. It is at this time that the continuous oscilloscopic display of the dynamic blood pressure comes into its own. The distal clamps on the common iliac arteries should be released such that one limb is opened at a time, allowing full time for all circulatory readjustments to settle before releasing the blood flow to the other limb. Whilst this is very straightforward with trouser-grafts, the surgeon may need reminding if a straight tube graft was all that was necessary. Again this problem is more severe in patients with aneurysms than in those with chronic occlusive aorto-iliac disease. Once the circulation is re-established to the lower limbs, the rate of blood transfusion is matched against the rate of blood loss from the anastomotic sites.

Haemostatic pause

Once all the major sites of haemorrhage have been dealt with, all the clamps have been released and the graft appears to be functioning well, there is not infrequently a period of oozing through the graft material (if a porous graft has been used), its anastomotic lines and suture holes. If the blood loss is not severe, it is worth asking the surgeon if he wishes to have a haemostatic pause. In this the anastomotic sites are packed with swabs, the wound lightly covered and the surgeon steps down from the operating table for ten minutes or so (he can usually be persuaded to have a cup of coffee then). In the meantime the anaesthetist keeps an eye on the various circulatory parameters and if these remain stable all is well. If the blood pressure starts to fall or if the rate of transfusion necessary to maintain the blood pressure starts to rise, the surgeon is alerted that there appears to be major bleeding from somewhere. Meanwhile the various minor oozing sites will have settled and clotted. The advantages of the haemostatic pause are that it enables the patient to readjust to the changes produced in his circulation in the absence of surgical stimuli, and any clotting is allowed to proceed without surgical disturbance. The sites of significant bleeding are then easily identified in the absence of the distraction of a general bleeding oozing. Finally, the graft, if it is going to clot off, will have done so by then, and this is very easy to identify. In practice it actually saves anaesthetic and operating time as, most commonly, the surgeon comes back to the operating table refreshed and when he removes the packs, he is confronted with a dry field so that he can then proceed briskly with wound closure. One other practical advantage accrues. It enables identification of the most common postoperative problems at the time that they are most likely to occur, viz, Has the graft clotted? and Is there any doubtful bleeding site? It may save a recall, perhaps late at night, when it has become manifestly obvious that re-exploration is necessary.

OTHER ASPECTS

There are a number of other aspects which, although applicable to most forms of surgery, yet are of particular importance during anaesthesia for vascular surgery.

Blood loss and blood transfusion

Few operations have such a variable demand for blood as operations on the aorta. This is due to the friable nature of the vessels, which can easily tear and the tear can run back to the renal arteries necessitating a quick suprarenal aortic clamping and a rapid suture of the tear, or even suturing the artery without clamping. The aneurysm itself may have evoked an inflammatory response so that the left common iliac vein has become densely adherent to the aneurysm, or the inferior vena cava can have become firmly attached to the wall of the aneurysm. Under such circumstances, the thin-walled veins can become easily damaged and require urgent repair. Meanwhile, there has been a sudden and severe blood loss. During the resection of the aneurysm there may be uncontrolled bleeding from the orifices of the lumbar arteries as they enter the posterior wall of the open aorta. There may be persistent oozing from the distal iliac vessels whose rigidity and calcification have deterred the surgeon from clamping too tightly for fear of cracking or splitting the whole vessel.

Blood and fluid balance need careful attention. It is good practice to weigh all the swabs after use and this, together with what has accumulated in the sucker bottle and with a generous allowance for the blood that has soaked into the drapes and surgeon's clothes, will provide a reasonably accurate estimate of the running total blood loss. This, though, is still second best to the careful observation of the arterial blood pressure and more importantly, the shape of the arterial blood pressure wave as displayed on the monitoring screen.

All the blood loss needs replacing and it is important not to get too far behind with the blood replacement, as in aortic surgery there is always the possibility of a sudden catastrophic haemorrhage occurring at any time, if only from the remote risk of an arterial clamp slipping. The rate of transfusion can vary from 0·5 l per hour up to 1 unit of blood per minute. Blood is normally cold and oesophageal temperature probes have shown that if the cold blood is transfused too quickly there can be a sharp fall in mid-oesophageal temperature, and so in the temperature of the heart. This will provoke a sharp fall in cardiac output, hypotension, bradycardia and severe dysrhythmias, which, in turn, can be misinterpreted as consequences of a severe haemorrhage and so more cold blood is given even more rapidly. It is important, therefore, that during aortic surgery all blood is given through a blood warmer, so that the blood is near normal body temperature before it enters the patient. Since both the timimg and the rate of transfusion are so unpredictable, the blood-warming apparatus should be set up as early as possible. It is important that the apparatus is capable of exchanging a large quantity of heat rapidly. Dipping a loop of the transfusion line into a bottle of warm water is hopelessly inadequate. Whether a dry blood warmer or a water bath is used is immaterial, but the efficiency of heat transfer should be such that blood flowing at a rate of 2 units per minute will be raised from refrigeration temperature to approximately 35 °C. The blood warmer should have several safety thermostats, two being barely adequate, and the control should be such that if the rate of transfusion is slowed down to a flow of 1 unit of blood per hour there will not be any over-heating of the blood. The principal danger is that the heater may contain hot spots which, at slow rates of transfusion, allow for localized over-heating. Dry heaters, unless great care has been taken in their design and manufacture, are more vulnerable in this respect.

Blood filters

Stored blood contains many micro-aggregates of blood debris. These can pass through the conventional Fenwall filter, with its 180 μ filter, which is the international standard for blood transfusion equipment. The micro-aggregates form a potent source of subsequent pulmonary problems by producing multiple small pulmonary emboli (Tomlin, 1976). The amount of micro-aggregates in one or two units of blood is of little importance, but if the transfusion is a large one the quantity of micro-aggregates becomes significant. Since the volume of blood transfusion is unpredictable, it is wiser to establish a fine blood filter right at the beginning rather than wait until it is clear that the transfusion is going to be a large one. It is then one less distraction to worry about when there is a sudden demand for rapid transfusion.

The pore size of the blood filter is of some practical significance, as the finer the pore size the more easily the filter clogs up. When the micro-aggregates reach the lung, they plug up the pulmonary arterioles. Each arteriole services approximately a dozen capillaries, and therefore, the same number of pulmonary alveolae. The average diameter of the pulmonary arteriole is slightly greater than 40 μ. Whilst loss of individual pulmonary capillaries is of no significance, the loss of a number of pulmonary arterioles can be of major significance. It is therefore logical to filter the blood down to 40 μ but not beyond this. The use of big bulky filters is not as helpful as would first seem, as the blood flow tends to channel through the filter (an analogy is the channelling which occurs when gases flow through the carbon dioxide absorber used in closed-circuit anaesthesia). In practical terms, filtering down to 40 μ enables up to 10 units of blood to be filtered at high flow rates before the filter clogs up with debris.

Accidental hypothermia

Anaesthesia for aortic surgery can be very prolonged. During this time the abdomen is opened and a large moist surface is exposed, ideal for surface evaporation of body water, and with that a loss of body heat. During anaesthesia the metabolic rate falls so that heat generation declines. In addition, the muscle relaxants inactivate a potential powerful heat source whilst the anaesthetic causes the body's thermoregulatory mechanism to go into abeyance. Heat becomes, therefore, more evenly distributed throughout the body so that the skin temperature rises whilst the core temperature falls. With the rise in skin temperature the radiant heat loss increases. Eventually, the skin temperature will fall, *pari passu*, with the core temperature. Thereafter, the body temperature falls remorselessly. Temperatures as low as 30 °C are now a distinct possibility whilst temperatures as low as 28·9 °C are not unknown. The temperature at which ventricular fibrillation occurs is 20 °C for the very young rising to 28 °C for the adult, but if the patient has ischaemic heart disease the temperature threshold for ventricular fibrillation can be higher. Before this stage is reached, there is a progressive fall in cardiac output (there is an exponential relationship between the reduction in size of the cardiac output and the degree of hypothermia, at 10%/ °C). Bradycardia and hypotension then develop with all the risks which these bring in patients with arterial disease.

Immediately after the end of the anaesthetic thermoregulatory control is resumed. The patient increases his metabolic rate and heat production to restore normothermia. This greatly increases his demand for oxygen. The increase in metabolism can be greater than any oxygen supply so that an oxygen debt occurs. All this develops at a time when the patient's ability to pick up oxyen is impaired (VA/Q inequalities are still present) and at a time when postoperative diffusion hypoxia (Fink et al., 1954) is still occurring. The hypothermia itself delays full recovery from the anaesthetic and is a major cause of patient distress, disorientation and confusion in the first two hours after anaesthesia.

It is, therefore, very important to try to prevent any unintentional hypothermia. This is best achieved by means of a heated water underblanket. Electric underblankets are not so satisfactory in that they do have hot spots and the distribution of heat is not uniform. Furthermore, the spillage of fluids used for skin preparation, which may contain solvents, raises questions about the safety of electric underblankets, apart from any blood or other fluids that might soak through.

Patients with ischaemic vascular disease are often obese and have a poor skin circulation. This means that some of the areas in contact with the underblanket may have a poor blood supply which is being worsened by the compression caused by the patient's weight. The rate of heat removal from such areas is, therefore, very poor. If the contact temperature is too high, first degree burns may result. The probability of such a burn depends upon two things: the heating temperature and the rate of heat removal. The worse the rate of heat removal, the lower is the heating temperature required to produce a thermal injury. A heating temperature of 35–36 °C will not produce a thermal injury and is enough to compensate for most of the heat losses due to evaporation. With such a blanket it is rare for the vascular patient to sustain a fall in core temperature of more than 1–2 °C. For patient safety it is essential that the water blanket should have more than one safety cut-out thermostat.

At the end of the operation it is a useful practice to wrap the patient in a 'space' blanket (a thin, plastic-coated highly reflective sheet of foil) to minimize any radiant heat loss. This facilitates a quicker termination of any accidental hypothermia and adds materially to the patient's comfort. When the patient starts to sweat, then the blanket has done its job. If a heated water underblanket is not available for the operation, then wrapping the patient's torso and limbs with a 'space' blanket prior to skin preparation will make a small contribution to reducing hypothermia, as will persuading the surgeon to cover the exposed bowel with large warm wet packs and keeping such packs wet and warm. If the packs get cold, they will remove some heat by conduction, although the amount of heat lost by this is considerably less than that lost by evaporation. A better strategy is to persuade the surgeon to fold the reflected bowel and mesentery into a plastic bag before he starts operating on the exposed aorta.

Fluid loss

There are three major sources of fluid loss: surface evaporation, bowel sequestration and renal excretion. Up to 2 l of fluid can be lost into the exposed bowel before it becomes obvious to the naked eye. Fluid is constantly being secreted into the lumen of the bowel and is subsequently re-absorbed. The fluid turnover per day exceeds 20 l. Fluid absorption is a totally distinct operation from secretion and can fail independently of either secretion or bowel motility. It is the first of these three components of bowel activity to fail, as any sufferer of diarrhoea knows only too well. Thus the observation of visible peristalsis, of the exposed intestines, is no guarantee that fluid is not accumulating in the lumen of the bowel. It is sequestered there and will be returned to the circulation eventually, days later. The fluid lost there is isotonic and has virtually the same composition as extracellular fluid. The most readily available fluid that is nearest in composition to this is Hartmann's solution and it is logical to replace all simple fluid losses with this fluid and to let the kidneys resolve to final ionic balance.

Renal function

During the cross-clamping phase there is a considerable reduction in renal function. As has been mentioned in Chapter 1, there is some dispute as to the precise aetiology of this. Recent work (Gamulin et al., 1984) has shown that during the period of infrarenal cross-clamping renal blood flow is reduced by a third, whilst renal vascular resistance almost doubles. More importantly, these changes persisted for at least an hour after the cross-clamp had been released. There is a strong clinical impression that a good diuresis aids renal blood flow and, in particular, the distribution of the blood flow between the renal cortex and medulla. A renal diuresis is, therefore, to be encouraged. Many vascular surgery patients have a mild degree of renal failure. If renal perfusion is well maintained, there will be a continuous production of urine. Furthermore, a good flow of urine reduces the possibility of major renal failure. An optimum is 50 ml of urine per hour, and if the rate of urine production falls below this the patient should be given a small dose of a diuretic, such as 20–40 mg frusemide, after ensuring that the patient has had a significant infusion of crystalloid solution. Such an approach will minimize the risk of postoperative renal failure, a complication to which the patient undergoing aortic surgery is only too prone.

Acid–base balance

During surgery on the aorta the blood supply to a large proportion of the body mass is deliberately occluded, and occluded for a long time, yet when the vascular obstruction is released there is remarkably little disturbance of the acid–base balance. After 45 min of total vascular occlusion of the infrarenal aorta following restoration of normal blood flow, the average disturbance of acid–base balance is rarely more than 2–3 mmol base deficit (Johnstone et al., 1965). If the vascular occlusion is very much longer than this, the patient is more in danger of developing a crush syndrome, of muscle necrosis and myoglobinuria, than of developing a severe metabolic acidosis, providing there has been no hypotension. Both of these conditions have a common origin. In practice, the occurrence of a crush syndrome following vascular surgery is exceedingly rare (Goormaghtigh, 1947; Oliver et al., 1951), although it used to be common when the now-obsolete operation of combined bilateral iliac, femoral, popliteal disobliteration was practised. The major source of a crush syndrome in vascular surgery practice is after an emergency femoral embolectomy which has been performed too late.

The smallness of the size of the disturbance of the acid–base balance is often a source of surprise, but on reflection this should not be so. Although the extent of the size of the body mass that has been deprived of its blood supply for a substantial period of time would lead to an expectation of a severe metabolic acidosis, this does not develop because, during anaesthesia, this large body mass is, metabolically, at a very low ebb.

At rest the infrarenal portion of the aorta receives less than one-eighth of the cardiac output, although this proportion of the body mass has a capacity of accepting five times this flow and its vessels are, accordingly, normally large enough to accommodate such a large flow should the occasion warrant. This portion of the body is well away from the thermally active central core, so that its metabolic rate is lower than the average of the body. During anaesthesia the metabolic rate declines as part of the general sedation effect of anaesthetic drugs. The muscle relaxants, by reducing muscle tone (which is a source of heat production), further reduce the metabolic rate particularly of the legs, whilst the circulatory occlusion which forms part of the operation, of itself obstructs the flow of heat from the central core to the lower limbs. As a result the lower limbs become hypothermic. All this reduces the demand of the lower limbs for oxygen and so enables the limbs to survive despite a prolonged period of total ischaemia without developing a marked metabolic acidosis, and more importantly without developing a crush syndrome. Whilst under anaesthesia and the influence of muscle relaxants, these patients can withstand a considerably longer period of total ischaemia to the lower limbs than can the conventional trauma patient who has had the circulation to his legs cut off.

If the total occlusion time to both legs exceeds $1\frac{1}{2}$ hours, it is worth measuring the degree of metabolic acidosis some 10 or more minutes after the surgeon has restored the blood flow and after the acid metabolites have been washed out into the general circulation. If the degree of metabolic acidosis exceeds 4 mmol base deficit, it is worth correcting, otherwise the liver will correct it very quickly.

A greater indication for measuring the acid–base balance is if there has been any period of prolonged hypotension, as may happen when dealing with a ruptured aortic aneurysm or a dissecting aneurysm. Under these circumstances the disturbance of acid–base balance is much more likely to be greater than that resulting from any reasonable period of controlled circulatory occlusion of the infrarenal aorta. However, if the circulatory occlusion is above the renal vessels or the mesenteric vessels or even the coeliac axis, then metabolic acidosis could be a problem as these vessels serve metabolically very active tissues. Anything more than a minor degree of metabolic acidosis should be treated vigorously as cardiac output falls linearly with falls in pH (Tomlin, 1966). This fall in cardiac output could lead to further hypotension, and a worsening of the acidosis which leads to yet more reduction in cardiac output and so on. The end result is a vicious spiral from which it becomes more and more difficult to break clear.

REFERENCES

Akerblom O., de Verdier C. H., Garby L. et al. (1968) Restoration of defective oxygen transport function of stored red blood cells by the addition of inosine. *Scand. J. Clin. Lab. Invest.* **21**, 245

Allison S. P., Tomlin P. J. and Chamberlain M. J. (1969) Some effects of anaesthesia and surgery on carbohydrate and fat metabolism. *Br. J. Anaesth.* **41**, 588

Atkinson R. S., Rushman G. B. and Lee J. A. (eds.) (1982) Vagal reflex mechanisms. In: *Synopsis of Anaesthesia*, 9th edn., p. 819. Wright PSG, Bristol

Beecher H. K. (1956) Relationship of significance of wound to the pain experienced. *JAMA* **161**, 1609

Bonnet F., Harari A., Thibonnier M. et al. (1982) Suppression of ADH hypersecretion during surgery by extradural anaesthesia. *Br. J. Anaesth.* **54**, 29

Brown M. M., Wade P. P. H. and Marshall J. (1985) Fundamental importance of arterial oxygen content in the regulation of cerebral blood flow in man. *Brain* **108**, 81

Camporesi E. M. and Redick L. F. (1983) Clinical aspects of spinal narcotics. In: *Opiate Analgesia*, p. 57. Editor: Bullingham R. E. S. Saunders, London

Catling J. A., Pinto D. M., Jordan C., et al. (1980) Respiratory effects of analgesia after cholecystectomy. Comparison of continuous and intermittent papaveretum. *Br. Med. J.* **ii**, 478

Child C. S. and Kaufman L. (1985) Effects of intrathecal diamorphine on the adrenocortical, hyperglycaemic and cardiovascular responses to major colonic surgery. *Br. J. Anaesth.* **57**, 389

Christensen P., Brandt M. R., Rem J. et al. (1982) Influence of extradural morphine on the adrenocortical and hyperglycaemic response to surgery. *Br. J. Anaesth.* **54**, 23

Church J. J. (1979) Continuous narcotic infusion for the relief of postoperative pain. *Br. Med. J.* **i**, 977

Collins J. A. (1980) Abnormal hemoglobin–oxygen affinity and surgical hemotherapy. In: *Surgical hemotherapy, Bibl. Haemat.*, p. 46. Editors: Collins J. A. and Lundsgaard-Hansen P. Karger, Basel.

Coote J. H. and Crawford J. S. (1983) Relevant considerations of neuroanatomy and neuro-physiology. In: *Scientific Foundations of Obstetrics and Gynaecology*. Editor: Barnes J. Heinemann, London

Cousins M. J., Mather L. E., Glynn C. J. et al. (1977) Selective spinal analgesia. *Lancet* **i**, 1141

Crile G. W. (1913) The kinetic theory of shock and its prevention through anoci-association (Shockless operations). *Lancet* **ii**, 7

Daniel M. K., Bennett B., Dawson A. A. et al. (1986) Haemoglobin concentration and linear cardiac output, peripheral resistance and oxygen transport. *Br. Med. J.* **292**, 923

De Almeida A. J. M. P. (1975) Some effects of inspiratory flow patterns on blood gas exchange in artificial ventilation in anaesthesia. PhD thesis, University of Birmingham

Fink R., Carpenter S. L. and Holaday D. A. (1954) Diffusion anoxia during recovery from nitrous oxide/oxygen anaesthesia. *Fed. Proc.* **13**, 354

Gamulin Z., Forster A., Morel D. et al. (1984) Effects of infrarenal aortic cross-clamping on renal haemodynamics in humans. *Anesthesiology* **61**, 394

Ganong W. F. (1983) Length of systole and diastole. In: *Review of Medical Physiology*, 11th edn., p. 452. Lange Medical Publications, California

Geigy (1970) *Documenta Geigy Scientific Tables*. p. 557. Geigy, Basle

Geyer R. P. (1982) Oxygen transport in vivo by means of perfluorochemical preparations. *New Engl. J. Med.* **307**, 304

Gjessing J. and Tomlin P. J. (1979) Patterns of postoperative pain. *Anaesthesia* **34**, 624

Gjessing J. and Tomlin P. J. (1981) Postoperative pain control with intrathecal morphine. *Anaesthesia* **36**, 286

Goormaghtigh N. (1947) The renal arteriolar changes in the anuric crush syndrome. *Am. J. Pathol.* **23**, 513

Guyton A. C. (1981) Epicardial versus endocardial blood flow. Effect of intramyocardial pressure. In: *Textbook of Medical Physiology*, 6th edn., p. 299. Saunders, London

Hakanson E., Rutberg H., Jorfeldt L. et al. (1985) Effects of extradural morphine or bupivacaine on the metabolic response to upper abdominal surgery. *Br. J. Anaesth.* **57**, 394

Hasbrouk J. D. (1970) Morphine anaesthesia for open heart surgery. *Ann. Thorac. Surg.* **10**, 364

Hjortso N. C., Christensen N. J., Anderson J. et al. (1985) Effects of extradural administration of local anaesthetic agents and morphine on the urinary excretion of cortisol, catecholamines and nitrogen following abdominal surgery. *Br. J. Anaesth.* **57**, 400

Husemeyer R. P., O'Connor M. C. and Davenport H. T. (1980) Failure of epidural morphine to relieve pain in labour. *Anaesthesia* **35**, 161

Johnstone H., Lawson L. T. and Mucklow R. G. (1965) Metabolic changes after aorta-iliac occlusion. *Br. Med. J.* **ii**, 974

Jones P. M. (1983) Artificial blood. *Br. Med. J.* **i**, 246

Kaufman L. (1981) Intrathecal heroin. *Lancet* **ii**, 1341

Keele C. A., Neil E. and Joels N. (1982) Body water and body fluid. In: *Samson Wright's Applied Physiology*, 13th edn., p. 19. Oxford University Press, Oxford

Korinek A. M., Languille M., Bonnet T. et al. (1985) Effects of postoperative extradural morphine on ADH secretion. *Br. J. Anaesth.* **57**, 407

Long D. M. (1982) Fluorocarbons and synthetic bloods: capabilities and future use. In: *Pathophysiology and Techniques of Cardiopulmonary Bypass*, Vol. 1, p. 12. Editor: Utley J. Williams & Wilkins, Baltimore

Malins A. F. (1979) Pulmonary oedema following radiological investigation of patients with peripheral occlusive arterial disease: Adverse reactions to the contrast media. *Am. Heart. J.* **97**, 676

Mathews E. T. (1977) Preservatives in drugs. *Lancet* **i**, 1004

Mathews E. T. and Abrams L. (1980) Intrathecal morphine in open heart surgery. *Lancet* **ii**, 543

Messahel F. M. and Tomlin P. J. (1981) Narcotic withdrawal syndrome after administration of intrathecal morphine. *Br. Med. J.* **283**, 471

Milocco I., Lof B. A., William-Olsson G. et al. (1985) Left ventricular function during anaesthesia induction and sternotomy in patients with ischaemic heart disease. A comparison of six anaesthetic techniques. *Acta Anaesthesiol. Scand.* **29**, 241

Mitsuno T., Ohyanagi H. and Naito R. (1982) Clincial studies on a perfluorochemical whole blood substitute. *Ann. Surg.* **195**, 60

Mollison P. L. (ed.) (1983) Transfusion in oligaemia. In: *Blood Transfusion in Clinical Medicine,* 7th edn., p. 35. Blackwell Scientific Publications, Oxford

Oliver J., Macdowell M. and Tracey A. (1951) The pathogenesis of acute renal failure associated with traumatic and toxic injury, renal ischemia, nephrotoxic damage and the ischemuric episode. *J. Clin. Invest.* **30**, 1307

Paton W. D. M. and Payne J. P. (ed.) (1968) Control of pain. In: *Pharmacological Principles and Practice,* p. 94. Churchill, London

Pharmaceutical Codex (1979a) *Morphine,* p. 575. Pharmaceutical Society of Great Britain. Pharmaceutical Press, London

Pharmaceutical Codex (1979b) *Dextrans,* p. 256. Pharmaceutical Society of Great Britain. Pharmaceutical Press, London

Phillips G. and Tomlin P. J. (1977) Arterial oxygen tensions in elderly and injured elderly patients. *Br. J. Anaesth,* **49**, 514

Pirofsky B. (1953) The determination of blood viscosity by a method based on Poiseuille's law. *J. Clin. Invest.* **32**, 292

Ring J., Sharkoff D. and Richter W. (1980) Intravascular persistence of hydroxyethyl starch (HES) after serial granulocyte collections using HES in man. *Vox Sang.* **39**, 181

Rudowski W. and Kostrazewska E. (1976) Blood substitutes. *Ann. R. Coll. Surg. Engl.* **58**, 115

Rusy B. F. (1971) Evaluating myocardial contractility. *Anesthesiology* **35**, 328

Rutter P. C., Murphy F. and Dudley H. A. F. (1980) Morphine: controlled trial of different methods of administration for postoperative pain relief. *Br. Med. J.* **280**, 12

Schultze H. E. and Heremans J. F. (eds.) (1966) In: *Molecular Biology of Human Proteins with special reference to Plasma Proteins.* Elsevier, Amsterdam

Scott D. B. and McClure J. (1979) Selective epidural analgesia. Lancet **i**, 1410

Scrimshire D. A. and Tomlin P. J. (1973) Gas exchange during the initial stages of nitrous oxide uptake and elimination in a lung model. *J. Appl. Physiol.* **34**, 775

Srivastava S. (1982) Epidural buprenorphine for postoperative pain relief. *Anaesthesia* **37**, 699

Taylor P. (1980) Neuromuscular blocking agents. In: *Pharmacological Basis of Therapeutics,* 6th edn., p. 220. Editors: Goodman L. S., Gilman A. G. and Gilman A. Macmillan, New York

Tomlin P. J. (1966) Quantitative effects of changes in arterial pH and Paco₂ upon cardiac output during halothane anaesthesia in dogs. *J. Physiol.* **185**, 66P

Tomlin P. J. (ed.) (1976) In: *Fine Screen Filtration of Stored Blood.* Pall Biomedical, Portsmouth

Tomlin P. J. and Duck F. A. (1975) Transoesophageal aortovelography in man. *Can. Anaesth. Soc. J.* **22**, 561

Twigley A. J. and Hillman K. M. (1985) The end of the crystalloid era. A new approach to peri-operative fluid administration. *Anaesthesia* **40**: 860

Uvarov E. B., Chapman D. R. and Isaacs A. (1973) *Dictionary of Science.* Penguin Reference Books, Harmondsworth

Valleri C. R. and Hirsh N. M. (1969) Restoration in vivo, of erythrocyte adenosine, 2,3-diphosphoglycerate, potassium ion, and sodium ion concentrations following the transfusion of acid citrate dextrose stored human red blood cells. *J. Lab. Clin. Med.* **73**, 722

Valtis D. J. and Kennedy A. C. (1954) Defective gas transport function of stored red blood cells. *Lancet* **i**, 119

Walker W. F. (1982) Vascular disease of the lower limb: sympathectomy. In: *Essential Surgical Practice*, p. 754. Editors: Cuschieri A., Giles G. R. and Moossa A. R. Wright PSG, Bristol

Wall P. D. (1978) The gate control theory of pain mechanisms. An examination and re-statement. *Brain* **101**, 1

Wang J. K., Nauss L. A. and Thomas J. E. (1979) Pain relief by intrathecally applied opiates in man. *Anesthesiology* **50**, 149

Welchew E. A. (1983) On demand analgesia. *Anaesthesia* **38**, 19

Williams P. L. and Warwick R. (1980a) Plexuses of the autonomic system. In: *Gray's Anatomy*, 36th edn., p. 1132. Churchill Livingstone, London

Williams P. L. and Warwick R. (1980b) Dorsal root afferent fibres. In: *Gray's Anatomy*, 36th edn., p. 889. Churchill Livingstone, London

Yaksh T. L. (1981) Spinal opiate analgesia, characteristics and principles of action. *Pain* **11**, 293

Yates C. J. P., Berent A., Andrews V. et al. (1979) Increase in leg blood flow by normovolaemic haemodilution in intermittent claudication. *Lancet* **ii**, 166

CHAPTER 5

Ruptured Aortic Aneurysm

Few cases presenting for emergency surgery can be as dramatic or as challenging as a patient with a ruptured aortic aneurysm who arrives virtually pulseless and with no detectable blood pressure. As the anaesthetist, you are challenged to keep the patient alive and in good condition whilst extensive, traumatic and painful surgery is performed. At the other end of the scale, such patients can be remarkably well, capable of withstanding long journeys by ambulance or even an aircraft flight of 1000 km or more. And, of course, there are all grades in between these extremes. This has led to some debate as to the best management of these patients, whether to transfer them to specialist centres (Slaney et al., 1971), or to treat them locally (Cox and Ware, 1981). The reason for such a wide span lies in the nature of ruptured aortic aneurysms.

The first stage of rupture of the aorta occurs when the aneurysm undergoes an acute stretch and dilatation as the media constraining the aneurysm gives way. The patient, at this stage, complains of a severe backache as well as a painful pulsatile intra-abdominal swelling. The aneurysm is held together only by the adventitia, the retroperitoneal tissues and the posterior peritoneum. This period can last for several days or it may only last a few minutes. Then comes the stage when the adventitia gives way and there is leak of blood into the retroperitoneal tissues. This leakage is unpredictable both in size and rate of leakage. Finally, the posterior peritoneum gives way and there is frank haemorrhage into the peritoneal cavity. The only compressive force left then is the muscle tonus of the anterior abdominal wall acting on a very low intra-aortic blood pressure. Any increase in blood pressure or reduction in abdominal wall tonus will alter this pressure gradient and allow more bleeding into the peritoneal cavity. The resulting flow will further tear the aorta and the haemorrhage may become catastrophic or even terminal.

This sequence of pathophysiological changes dictates the optimum clinical management. Since the restraining tissues can give way at any time and progress to an uncontrolled haemorrhage, speed in initiating surgical treatment is essential. Delays in the anaesthetic room must be

146

avoided. Similarly, if the intraperitoneal pressure is reduced, as happens when a relaxant is given, the risk of uncontrollable haemorrhage increases substantially with every passing minute. In the final analysis when faced with a dire emergency case of ruptured aortic aneurysm, the anaesthetist can manage with one open vein and a finger on the radial pulse until such time as the surgeon has a crossclamp on the aorta above the aneurysm. The advantages of inserting a radial artery cannula, a central venous pressure monitoring line, an ECG and a blood pressure cuff, all before the surgery, are considerably outweighed by the disadvantages of the risk of an extension of the rupture in the wall of the aorta. The same argument applies to inserting a urinary bladder catheter under anaesthesia prior to starting surgery. If the catheter can be inserted quickly whilst preparing the skin and before the induction of anaesthesia, little is lost. The degree of urgency depends upon the state of the patient and, in particular, the extent of any hypotension.

The other aspect in the clinical management of patients presenting with a ruptured aortic aneurysm which needs to be considered is that these patients are emergency patients and are likely to have food and drink residues in their stomachs. There is no justification for any attempt to empty their stomachs preoperatively. The resulting straining may worsen the rupture of the aorta by transiently increasing the venous return to the left side of the heart, and so momentarily increasing the cardiac output and blood pressure, which would put further mechanical stress on the damaged part of the aorta. This aspect of straining also applies to the act of intubation and points to the need to maintain total paralysis once the trachea has been intubated. Straining and bucking on the endotracheal tube should be avoided if at all possible.

Wyatt (1976) describes five crisis points in the management of ruptured aortic aneurysms. These are (a) before the start of the anaesthetic, (b) anaesthetic induction, (c) decompression problems on opening the abdomen, (d) aortic clamp release, (e) postoperative oozing.

The anaesthetic requirement, therefore, is for a very rapidly acting induction agent followed by a muscle relaxant, which produces total and complete paralysis and in a dose that covers the merging period as a second longer-acting but slower-onset muscle relaxant takes over. This second relaxant should immediately follow the short-acting relaxant. The choice of induction agent, provided that it is of very rapid onset, is probably of less importance than the anaesthetist's familiarity with all the possible idiosyncrasies of the agent. When dealing with a potential ruptured aortic aneurysm patient, there is no place for trying out an unfamiliar induction agent. Otherwise, if there is an unexpected or untoward response, the distraction occasioned by wondering if it was due to the unfamiliar induction agent may delay the institution of corrective therapy appropriate to the true case. Tubocurarine should not be chosen for the long-acting muscle relaxant because of its ganglion blocking powers (Taylor, 1980), which will abolish any active vasoconstricting mechanisms.

Once the quick-acting relaxant has been given, then due to the hazards of a blowback from what might be a pressurized full stomach, no attempt should be made to ventilate the patient via a face mask prior to intubation. If there is time, oxygenation should be ensured by establishing a good reservoir of oxygen in the lungs by pre-oxygenation prior to intubation. This is followed by a 'crash' or rapid sequence induction technique using the minimum dose of any convenient rapidly acting induction agent as the circulating blood volume must be presumed to have been substantially reduced. Then succinyl choline is given and cricoid pressure is applied as soon as consciousness is lost. If the cricoid pressure makes intubation difficult, it is better to abandon this in order to facilitate a speedy intubation.

As soon as the trachea is intubated and if the pulse pressure fades at this point, the surgeon is alerted and told to start, whilst the anaesthetist relies on the anaesthesia produced by the induction agent. The surgeon must get his cross-clamp on the aorta as fast as possible otherwise there may be a cardiac arrest. This fall in pulse pressure can be due to one of two causes: (a) the induction agent has depressed a highly active compensatory vasoconstriction mechanism that was sustaining some form of circulation to the essential organs, or (b) the muscle relaxation has lowered the abdominal wall muscle tone so that all compressive forces on the posterior peritoneum are lost and so this peritoneum gives way and the aneurysm is bleeding into the peritoneal cavity. If the pulse pressure remains good, a slightly, but only very slightly, more leisurely approach may be used, i.e. inflate the endotracheal tube cuff and secure the tube and then get some nitrous oxide into the lungs before the surgeon starts his incision. The circulating blood volume should be expanded as fast as possible, ideally with whole blood but any intravenous fluid will do, in order to compensate for any loss of vasoconstrictor tone produced by the induction agent. Although any intravenous fluid will do, if there is no blood or PPF immediately available, the gelatin solutions are the best first choice. At this stage the patient is very lightly anaesthetized and the sympathetic stimulation produced by the skin incision will stimulate the vasomotor centre and overcome any depression produced by the induction agent. Once the aorta has been cross-clamped, then attention can be given to establishing the various monitoring lines and the resuscitation completed.

Thus, the practical aspects of the initial management can be summarized as follows. All anaesthetic drugs are prepared and drawn up in their respective syringes. An open vein is secured and the patient placed on the operating table with an arm abducted. (This is for subsequent arterial cannulation.) The bladder is quickly catheterized providing that the patient is not too hypotensive and the skin prepared for surgery. An intravenous fluid infusion is started through the open vein. Meanwhile, the patient is given oxygen to breathe. An assistant or nurse monitors the pulse continuously. If there is time, ECG contacts are stuck onto the skin. When the abdomen is completely draped and the surgeon scrubbed and ready, the anaesthetic is started using the rapid-sequence induction technique. The induction agent, short-acting and longer-acting muscle relaxants are given in quick succession. If the pulse fades, the surgeon is told to proceed quickly and the infusion rate increased. The ventilator is connected, endotracheal tube cuff inflated, the tube is secured and the patient placed on a ventilator, to be ventilated with a 50 : 50 nitrous oxide–oxygen mixture until the aorta is cross-clamped.

Once the aorta is cross-clamped, the anaesthetic can be deepened, if necessary, with an intravenous narcotic. Morphine produces the least disturbance of the circulation, pethidine the most, with fentanyl and phenoperidine lying in between. If the blood pressure is stable and if fentanyl or phenoperidine has been used, then droperidol can be given. Droperidol has mild adrenergic alpha-receptor blocking powers and if the patient has an unstable circulation very severe hypotension will result. The droperidol will potentiate the analgesic properties of phenoperidine or fentanyl and even out the swinging of the depth of anaesthesia that occurs as either of these two drugs starts to lose its effect. Although intrathecal or epidural narcotics produce better analgesia, they have no place in the anaesthetic management of a potentially ruptured aortic aneurysm. The delays occasioned by this technique are unwarranted, whilst the positioning of the patient may cause the acutely dilated aneurysm to rupture into the peritoneal cavity.

Arterial cannulation is best performed once the aorta has been cross-clamped and the anaesthetic stabilized. It should not be performed under local anaesthesia with the patient conscious, neither should the operation be delayed whilst the anaesthetist inserts the arterial cannula. If the patient is hypotensive this can make arterial cannulation very difficult. More importantly, during the time taken to set up this line the aneurysm may give way, catastrophically. The rise in blood pressure which often occurs when the clamp is applied will facilitate the actual arterial cannulation. Thereafter the general principles of management for an elective resection of an aneurysm that were described in Chapter 4 now apply, but the patient still requires above-average vigilance.

BLOOD SUBSTITUTES IN BLOOD LOSS

If, after cross-clamping the aorta, the arterial pressure is still low, the patient will need a very rapid blood transfusion immediately. Blood substitutes will suffice for the first litre of resuscitation, but thereafter they are progressively of less and less value. If cross-matched blood is still not available then group O Rhesus negative unmatched blood should be used. If this is not available in sufficient quantity, then group O Rhesus positive blood should be used. Rarely, it may be necessary to use blood that has only been group matched, but this may create problems, particularly among group A recipients.

The reason why after only a litre or so of blood substitutes they become progressively of less value lies in the oxygen flux—that is, how much oxygen is flowing into the aorta. It is the product of cardiac output, haemoglobin saturation and haemoglobin concentration, as was discussed in Chapter 1 (p. 28). In the case of the ruptured aortic aneurysm with a low blood pressure the cardiac output is reduced because the venous return is reduced. The venous return is particularly depleted of oxygen (normally the venous return has a 75% load of oxygen; Ganong 1983). Its transit time through the lung is particularly fast, and so it does not pick up all the oxygen it could carry. If blood is 75% desaturated, it takes approximately 0·1 s for the blood to become fully saturated with oxygen (Nunn, 1981a; Keele et al., 1982a). In normal health the transit time of blood to cross the alveolae is about 0·8 s so there is a reasonable reserve of time (Staub et al., 1962). If the venous blood is below 50% saturated it takes 0·2 s or more to become fully saturated with oxygen (Nunn, 1981b). (If the venous return is low because of loss of circulating blood volume, what little blood that remains is pumped around faster and faster among the essential organs which in turn extract more and more oxygen.) In addition, in hypovolaemia there is a marked ventilation–perfusion ratio inequality as well as a marked increase in physiological deadspace (sometimes this part of the physiological deadspace is called the 'parallel' deadspace, for obvious reasons; Folkow and Pappenheimer, 1955). Together these also contribute to the hypoxaemia. Increasing the circulating blood volume with blood substitutes improves the venous return, improves the ventilation–perfusion ratio defect and increases the transit time across the pulmonary alveolae. To that end arterial oxygenation is improved. The arterial tension and so the arterial oxygen saturation rise, but the blood is thinner. Once near full saturation is achieved, the limiting factor on the oxygen supply is the haemoglobin concentration. Diluting the blood further will have no effect—apart from the trivial case of increasing the amount of physical solution available for dissolving in simple solution. The effects can be seen in the following example.

Let the initial haemoglobin be 15 g% and cardiac output be 5 l/min, and the liver blood supply be 1·5 l/min. This initial situation is a healthy one, being situation (a) in *Table* 5.1.

Now let there be a haemorrhage so that the cardiac output falls by 40% to 3 l/min. The liver is an essential organ and its blood supply only falls by 27% to 1·1 l/min, but because of the oxygenation problems within the pulmonary circulation the arterial oxygen saturation has fallen to 90%. This is situation (b) in *Table* 5.1.

Now let 1 l of blood substitute be given. The cardiac output rises to 4 l/min, the haemoglobin has to fall to 11·25 g%, but the oxygenation problems improve somewhat to a saturation of 97% and the liver blood flow improves to 1·3 l/min (i.e. cardiac output is still down by 20% but liver flow is down only 14%). This is situation (c) in *Table* 5.1.

Finally, a second litre of blood substitute is given which restores all flows to normal including cardiac output and liver flow. Arterial oxygen saturation is also normal, but the haemoglobin must fall to 9·0 g%. This is situation (d) in *Table* 5.1.

Table 5.1 Oxygen flux and liver oxygen supply after haemorrhage and with replacement by blood substitutes

Situation	Cardiac output (ml/min)	Hb (g%)	Saturation (%)	O_2 flux (ml/min)
(a) Healthy	5000	15	98	985
(b) 2 litres loss	3000	15	90	543
(c) +1 litre PPF	4000	11.25	97	585
(d) +2 litres PPF	5000	9	98	590

Liver Oxygenation Situation	Blood flow (ml/min)	Hb (g%)	Saturation (%)	O_2 Supply (ml/min)
(a)	1500 (100%)	15	98	295
(b)	1100 (73%)	15	90	200
(c)	1300 (86%)	11.25	97	190
(d)	1500 (100%)	9	98	177

It is possible to calculate the oxygen flux and the oxygen supply to the liver for all similar situations. While these figures can only be rough approximations, it will be seen that increasing the venous return by the use of a blood substitute to below the normal venous return improves the oxygen output from the heart, whilst having a negligible effect on the oxygen supply to the liver, or for that matter, any of the other vital organs. If, however, the full severe blood loss is replaced with blood substitute, there is little further improvement of the oxygen output from the heart and, more importantly, some of the diminished oxygen supply is diverted away from the vital organs to go to non-essential tissues. If there is mechanical obstruction to the arterial supply of an essential organ, such as a patch of atheroma in a coronary vessel, the improvement in arterial blood pressure following the infusion of blood substitute, together with the reduced viscosity of the blood produced by the blood substitute, could enable the diluted blood to be squeezed past the patch of atheroma thereby increasing the oxygen supply to that particular organ.

In any severe circulatory shutdown situation which is due to haemorrhage, the reduction in blood flow to the local tissues is mediated mainly by throttling back the inflow to those tissues by arteriolar vasoconstriction. There is, in addition, another mechanism whereby tissues are deprived of blood flow. This is by opening arteriolar–venous shunts. These shunts occur immediately distal to the arteriole. The skin is well endowed with them (Keele et al., 1982b), but other tissues also have them. Their effects are twofold: a conserving of tissue oxygen uptake so that the venous blood is not quite so desaturated as it could be, and a quickening of the venous return as the transit time through the precapillary shunt is much less than the transit time through the capillaries. But it does mean that some of the reduced oxygen flux is unused and this must represent inefficiency and wasted effort. Improving the flow, even with diluted blood, to any tissue reduces the precapillary shunt effect and makes the circulatory system that much more efficient. Whether this is of immediate benefit to the patient or not depends upon whether the tissue concerned was a vital one or not.

These benefits may be long-term or short-term. The body's compensatory circulatory defence mechanisms work only for the short-term benefit and long-term needs receive short shrift. The most important example is the kidneys, which are rich in arteriovenous anastomoses. If there is a reduction in renal blood flow consequent upon a fall in cardiac output the reduction in renal parenchymal flow is mediated, in part, by vasoconstriction and in part by the opening of these shunts. The reduced parenchymal blood flow may precipitate cellular death or acute renal tubular necrosis. Expanding the flow, even with blood substitutes, such as PPF, reduces this shunt flow, thereby increasing the supply of oxygen to the kidney parenchymal cells. In effect the treatment has over-ridden the body's view that the kidneys are a non-vital organ.

Thus, expanding an acutely depleted circulating blood volume with plasma or blood substitute can lead to the prevention of such long-term consequences as renal failure by improving not only the net efficiency of the oxygen uptake at the periphery but also to a more equitable distribution of oxygen to the tissues. There is a limit and with a haemoglobin concentration much below 60–70%, i.e. a haemoglobin concentration of less than 10 g%, the disadvantages outweigh the advantages.

This point has been laboured since when faced with a patient with a ruptured aortic aneurysm, the relatively ready availability of blood substitutes as compared with the difficulty and delays in obtaining sufficient quantities of cross-matched blood may lead to a temptation to use too much blood substitute.

INTRA-OPERATIVE CARE

Once the anaesthesia is established, the abdomen opened and the aorta cross-clamped the immediate crisis is over. The anaesthetist can now establish his various monitoring aids, particularly the arterial line. A central venous pressure line is an additional convenience for the anaesthetic, but no more than that, although it could be very useful postoperatively. Nevertheless, these patients still require above-average vigilance by the anaesthetist. The circulating blood volume still needs to be restored as quickly as possible to minimize the possibility of either a myocardial infarction or renal tubular necrosis. The rate of urinary output needs close attention. If the urine production relative to the blood pressure falls below 0·5 ml/min the patient should be given a rapidly acting diuretic, such as frusemide. The dose required should be that which would produce a diuresis in a patient with presumed reasonably normal kidneys; 20–40 mg should suffice even though the patient is likely to be elderly with a mild degree of chronic renal failure. If this fails to produce a response, the dose should be doubled or even trebled, as it must be presumed that there is some degree of acute tubular necrosis.

Part of this judgement is the urinary output relative to the blood pressure. It is highly unlikely that the patient's true blood pressure will be known. By virtue of the presenting problem it must be assumed that the patient has widespread arterial disease and therefore that the blood pressure is normally raised. There are some indicators which would suggest that the pressure should be very high, i.e. that this particular patient should have a systolic blood pressure of around 200 mmHg. These indicators are the shape of the arterial pressure wave, and in particular, the presence of multiple dichrotic notches, and the calibre and texture of the radial artery on palpation. If it is thick and hard, it is likely that the systolic pressure should be raised. Other pointers are a raised diastolic pressure, evidence of left ventricular hypertrophy on the ECG or splitting or notching of the QRS wave of the ECG.

If, at operation, the aorta is found to have leaked or ruptured into the retroperitoneal tissues, there will subsequently be a lot of exudate into those tissues. Exudate is rich in protein and so the patient will need, in addition to blood, an infusion of plasma or PPF. There are no firm guidelines on how much to give or how much is needed, but empirically a ratio of 1 unit of PPF to 5 units of whole blood seems to give the best chance of achieving haemodynamic stability.

The patient is likely to have been under-perfusing his tissues for a period of time. Once the circulating blood volume has been restored, it is worth obtaining an assessment of the acid–base status. Unless the patient has been very hypotensive for a very long period of time, it is not worth measuring the acid–base status until the circulating blood volume has been restored, as any result will be an under-estimate of the true severity of the acidosis. Whilst the patient is hypovolaemic, acid metabolites will be accumulating in the under-perfused non-essential tissues. These acids will not find their way into the circulation until normovolaemia has been restored. It is more logical to assume that there is a degree of metabolic acidosis and to give 100 mmol of sodium bicarbonate with calcium chloride cover as part of the resuscitation. Then, when normovolaemia has been achieved, the degree of metabolic acidosis is measured in order to determine how much further alkali will be necessary to achieve acid–base balance. With very severe hypotension this rough empirical approach is likely to be insufficient, and it is likely that 200 or more mmol of bicarbonate may be necessary. This cannot be predicted so it is better to measure the acid–base status after fluid resuscitation has started, even though the answer is very likely to be an under-estimate of the true position. If the blood pressure and cardiac output during the operation are unstable, then there is likely to be yet further under-perfusion and so further acidosis. Under such circumstances repetitive estimations of the acid–base status should be made.

These patients are very high risk patients. Whilst the mortality from elective resection of an aortic aneurysm is about 4%, with the urgent but unruptured aneurysms (acute stretch group) the mortality varies from 6% to 36%. In contrast, if the aneurysm has frankly ruptured the mortality varies from 40% to 69% (Hicks et al., 1975). Gore and Hirst (1973) in an analysis of 46 published reports involving 1516 patients found that the average mortality was 54%. These numbers refer to those who got as far as the anaesthetic room. Obviously some of the frankly ruptured group die *en route*. Without surgery the mortality is 100%, including the acute stretch group since they will rupture very soon. Apart from the time and effort, there is nothing lost in trying to save these patients. Some of the patients inevitably will have suffered some degree of myocardial damage as a result of this acute episode. This will show as a persistently low blood pressure and cardiac output despite vigorous resuscitation efforts. The presence of engorged neck veins, or if there has been time to establish a central venous pressure line a raised central venous pressure, strongly suggest that there is some degree of reduced myocardial contractility. If at this stage no alkali has yet been given, then some should be given rather quickly. If there is still no improvement, then a bolus dose of 5 mmol of calcium ions should be given. If there is still no response it is likely that the myocardial damage is severe and may be permanent. If there is a flicker of response, then the outlook is that much more favourable. Either way, the calcium ions should be followed by a dilute infusion of inotropic drugs such as isoprenaline or an isoprenaline–adrenaline mixture. In some patients the improvement in circulatory haemodynamics produced by the calcium ions alone may be enough, in which case the prognosis is even better. There still will be a small hard core of patients in whom nothing is capable of inducing a response. The damage is too severe. The outlook for these particular patients is then very bad. Some will die on the operating table, while others will survive for a variable period in the intensive care unit only to peter out with renal failure or even multiple systems failure. Occasionally, though, one can be surprised in that after a period of being totally refractory to all drugs, the circulation gradually picks up and after a stormy and protracted period of very intensive after-care, complete with haemodialysis, the patient slowly improves to be eventually discharged from hospital. Such cases are clinically very satisfying but very rare.

Apart from these points, the patient with a ruptured aortic aneurysm is treated during the anaesthetic period much like any other case of aortic aneurysm.

POSTOPERATIVE CARE

If at operation the aorta was frankly ruptured with either an intraperitoneal haemorrhage or a large retroperitoneal haematoma, then immediately after operation it is important to maintain artificial ventilation for at least 16 hours postoperatively. There is likely to be much retroperitoneal oedema and tension. This is a source of much postoperative pain. It induces inefficient ventilation and so increases the disturbance of the ventilation–perfusion ratio. There is a very marked difference in the severity of the alveolar–arterial oxygen tension differences between those patients who have had a frank rupture and those whose problem was an acute dilatation and stretching of the lower aorta without rupture. The patient with frank rupture has a much more severe postoperative hypoxaemia and it persists for a much longer period of time. More significant is the fact that the ventilation–perfusion ratio disturbance intensifies postoperatively to reach a maximum at about 12–18 hours after the end of operation. At about this time, if the patient has been allowed to breathe on his own, the hypoxaemia may be so severe that the patient goes into frank respiratory failure. Yet up to this time the same patient may have appeared to be so well, with a good circulation, blood pressure and reasonable blood gas values, that the attending staff in the intensive care unit have fallen into the trap of allowing spontaneous ventilation and extubating the patient. A few hours later the hypoxaemia declares itself. It the patient has been prematurely discharged from the intensive care unit to the ward delays, in recognition of this hypoxaemia problem, coupled with delays in getting the patient re-admitted to the intensive care unit, may precipitate a hypoxaemic emergency. On re-admission to the intensive care unit the patient will need artificial ventilation and intensive pulmonary physiotherapy for several days.

The patients with a major retroperitoneal haematoma are also likely to develop a severe paralytic ileus. This takes up to 16 hours to declare itself and the resulting mechanical distension of the abdomen will further add to the respiratory difficulties, and indeed is one of the indications for artificial ventilation in these patients. The ileus will cause significant shifts of water between the various fluid compartments of the body and can precipitate delayed renal failure.

It is, therefore, essential in the management of all patients who have had a ruptured aortic aneurysm which has caused a major retroperitoneal haematoma that they remain in an intensive care unit for at least 36 hours after the operation, and that considerable attention is directed at their oxygenation and urinary output throughout all this time. At the slightest indication of a fall in urinary output a forced diuresis should be maintained with, if need be, large doses of diuretic. Renal failure after ruptured aortic aneurysm is very common (Abbott and Beck, 1975). The anaesthetist can make a valuable contribution in preventing this by minimizing or preventing any severe hypotension. Nevertheless, in those hospitals that have vascular surgery units, a common reason for emergency haemodialysis is renal failure following surgical correction of a ruptured aortic aneurysm. Furthermore, these patients are not usually suitable for subsequent kidney transplantation if there is permanent severe kidney damage.

REFERENCES

Abbott W. M. and Beck C. H. (1975) Renal failure after ruptured aneurysm. *Arch. Surg.* **110**, 1110

Cox R. and Ware C. C. (1981) Abdominal aneurysms in a district general hospital. *Ann. R. Coll. Surg. Engl.* **63**, 177

Folkow B. and Pappenheimer J. R. (1955) Components of the respiratory deadspace and their variation with pressure breathing and with broncho-active drugs. *J. Appl. Physiol.* **8**, 102

Ganong W. F. (1983) Gas transport between the lung and the tissues. In: *Review of Medical Physiology*, 11th edn., p. 533. Lange Medical Publications, Chicago

Gore I. and Hirst A. E. (1973) Arteriosclerotic aneurysms of the abdominal aorta, a review *Prog. Cardiovasc. Dis.* **16**, 113

Hicks G. L., Eastland M. W., DeWeese J. A. et al. (1975) Survival improvement following aortic aneurysm resection. *Ann. Surg.* **181**, 863

Keele C. A., Neil E. and Joels N. (1982a) Kinetics of the reaction between oxygen and haemoglobin. In: Samson Wright's Applied Physiology, 13th edn., p. 186. Oxford University Press, Oxford

Keele C. A., Neil E. and Joels N. (1982b) Circulation through special regions. In: *Samson Wright's Applied Physiology*, 13th edn., p. 133. Oxford University Press, Oxford

Nunn J. F. (ed.) (1981a) Kinetics of the reaction of oxygen with haemoglobin. In: *Applied Respiratory Physiology*, 2nd edn., p. 404. Butterworth, London

Nunn J. F. (ed.) (1981b) Changes in Po_2 in the pulmonary capillary. In: *Applied Respiratory Physiology*, 2nd edn., p. 317. Butterworth, London

Slaney G., Ashton F., Barnes A. D. et al. (1971) Management of aortic aneurysms. *Br. Med. J.* **ii**, 525

Staub N. C., Bishop J. M. and Forster R. E. (1962) Importance of diffusion and the chemical reaction rates in oxygen uptake in the lungs. *J. Appl. Physiol.* **17**, 21

Taylor P. (1980) Neuromuscular blocking agents. In: *Pharmacological Basis of Therapeutics*, 6th edn., p. 220. Editors: Goodman L. S., Gilman A. G. and Gilman A. Macmillan, New York

Wyatt A. P. (1976) Presentation and management of aneurysms. *Ann. R. Coll. Surg. Engl.* **58**, 52

CHAPTER 6

Carotid Artery Surgery

PHYSIOLOGICAL ASPECTS

Modern carotid artery surgery started in 1954 with the first report of a successful carotid endarterectomy (Eastcott et al., 1954). Since that time the operation has been adopted world wide. The commonest indication is to reduce, if not abolish, attacks of transient cerebral ischaemia that herald the possibility of a major cerebral infarction. The commonest site of the arterial occlusion or stenosis is at the bifurcation of the common carotid artery and this is treated by endarterectomy at that site. If the arterial obstruction within the internal carotid is more extensive, a recent development is to make an anastomosis between the external carotid artery circulation and a surface vessel on the cerebral cortex through a small craniotomy. However, the anaesthetic requirements for both operations are very similar.

Compared with other types of vascular surgery that for the carotid artery poses quite different problems for the anaesthetist. The loss of large volumes of blood during this type of surgery is rare and there are negligible changes in the size of the vascular bed during the operative period, despite the clamping of the carotid artery. Indeed, it is one of the surgeon's objectives to maintain the cerebral perfusion as little changed as possible during the operation. The brain normally receives about 750 ml blood per minute and during the surgery this flow is maintained either through the remaining cerebral vessels via their anastomoses in the circle of Willis or by the surgeon deliberately inserting a temporary plastic shunt in the vessel on which he is working.

During anaesthesia cerebral blood flow is critically dependent upon three things: (a) the arterial blood pressure, (b) the blood gases and (c) the presence of volatile anaesthetic agents.

Although the intracranial vessels are well endowed with both adrenergic and cholinergic nerves (Iwayama et al., 1970), the cerebral vessels have very few active sympathetic nerve fibres supplying them.

Within the cerebral vessels the resting sympathetic tone is minimal, although the cerebral vasculature is richly innervated by branches from the superior cervical ganglia. The role of these sympathetic nerves in the regulation of cerebral blood flow is unclear (Heistad and Kontos, 1983), although it must be presumed that they protect the cerebral microvasculature and cerebrospinal fluid forming tissues against the effects of sudden surges in blood pressure. The overwhelming majority of the active nerve fibres supplying the head travel with the external carotid artery. Those destined for the arterioles then travel with the various branches of that artery, including those anastomotic vessels that pierce the skull, and link the external and internal carotid circulations, such as the middle meningeal–ophthalmic arterial anastomoses. These diploeic vessels are only capable of supplying the cerebral cortex to a depth of 1 cm or less. The extent of this is very variable between patients. The sympathetic fibres which accompany the diploeic vessels also supply the sympathetic nerves to the dura, as every migraine sufferer is only too aware. This accounts for the focal cortical ischaemia that may be identified on an EEG during an attack of migraine, or the general reduction in cortical blood flow seen in the aura phase of such an attack (O'Brien, 1967). Apart from the fibres which accompany the diploeic vessels, there are no sympathetic vasodilator fibres inside the skull. Hence any fall in blood pressure cannot be compensated for by local active vasodilatation. More than in any other tissue, the cerebral blood flow is dependent upon the driving blood pressure. Thus those drugs or anaesthetic agents which act primarily on the sympathetic nervous system have very little direct effect upon cerebral blood flow, although indirectly, via their effects upon the blood pressure, cerebral blood flow may be very considerably disturbed.

The cerebral vessels have an intrinsic auto-regulatory control mechanism which is sensitive to the internal distending pressure (Keele et al., 1982). The mechanism by which this operates is obscure, and it is a slowly adaptive one. It can be overwhelmed, as in malignant hypertension, where the excess pressure leads to cerebral oedema and papilloedema. The mechanism operates to maintain a reasonably constant cerebral perfusion irrespective of the long-term changes in the blood pressure. Thus the patient with chronic hypertension has the same cerebral blood flow as the normotensive patient. Between different species the mean arterial pressure within the brain is remarkably constant and lies between 70 and 90 mmHg despite wide variations in hydrostatic load between different species. One has only to consider the giraffe which has the same mean intracranial blood pressure as man and is capable of maintaining this whether the head is raised, as the animal forages for leaves at the top of an acacia tree, or the head is lowered, as the animal dips its head down to a pool of water for a drink (Warren, 1974). In man, too, whether lying down or standing up cerebral blood flow is unchanged.

At the lower end of the arterial pressure range, if the driving pressure is too low, the cerebral perfusion will fall notwithstanding all attempts of the auto-regulatory control mechanisms to dilate and to improve flow. The compensating mechanisms start to fail at a pressure of approximately 60–70 mmHg when cerebral perfusion starts to fall off (Harper, 1966), but severe brain damage is unlikely above an arterial blood pressure of 25 mmHg in a normotensive subject (Selkoe and Myers, 1979). The compensatory mechanisms also come into play with the hypertensive patient without arteriosclerosis, although the 'safety level' of pressure is not known. If there is marked obstructive atherosclerosis, cerebral function will deteriorate at a higher pressure depending upon the degree of partial vascular obstruction. It is important to appreciate that failure of neuronal function is not synonymous with neuronal cell death, although it is a stage on the way to cell death. Failure of cerebral function with severe hypotension is more or less constant across the whole of the cerebral cortex, whereas brain stem function persists until the pressure is very much lower. This has some practical application for the anaesthetist when monitoring the EEG during anaesthesia. Precise placing of the EEG electrodes is not critical in determining whether there is any failing of cerebral function, although, clearly, during carotid artery surgery the EEG electrodes should be placed over the field supplied by the relevant carotid artery.

There is a paradox between the uniformity of failure of cerebral function and the vulnerability of different areas of the brain to ischaemia, localized anoxia and neuronal death. Thus the occipital cortex, followed by the temporal lobes, is more vulnerable than the motor cortex (Stephenson, 1974). The cerebellum is more resistant whilst the brain stem is relatively robust. Hence, if as a result of ischaemia or anoxia there is brain stem death, it may be safely concluded that the cerebral cortex is dead, even though the reverse is not true (Tomlin et al., 1981).

The different parts of the brain have markedly different flow rates (Sokoloff and Kety, 1960) with the reticular formation having the highest flow rate and the corpus callosum having the lowest (Landau, 1955). The auto-regulatory control mechanism, which maintains optimum blood flow within the brain and the various parts of the brain despite changes in blood pressure, operates at the arteriolar level. The smooth muscle of the arteriole responds critically and sensitively not only to any accumulation of locally produced metabolites but also to its own intramural pressure, constricting when subject to a high distending force or relaxing when the distending force falls. This smooth muscle is markedly affected by volatile inhalational agents, notably halothane (McDowell, 1965). Halothane very markedly increases cerebral blood flow, and this increase occurs at very low concentrations, as low as 0·25%. This does have some practical significance in the vascular surgery patient. During carotid angiography, if halothane is being given, the velocity of the blood flow and the transit time of the contrast medium may be so fast that a small intracranial aneurysm may not be delineated. It will throw out all the timing calculations of the various phases of cerebral perfusion—the arterial filling phase, the capillary flush, the venous phase, etc.—for the different film exposures. Repeated radiological exposures may then be needed and the anaesthetic is unduly and unnecessarily prolonged. This is not as academic as it first appears. If the aneursym is in that part of the brain supplied by the diseased carotid artery, then the surgical reconstruction of the carotid artery will expose the aneurysm to the full force of the systolic blood pressure perhaps for the first time, with potentially disastrous results. At least one patient has died from this very cause, when a preoperative angiogram failed to delineate an intracranial aneurysm although it demonstrated flow through a stenosed carotid artery. The percentage of people with intracranial aneurysms has been variously estimated as between 0·1% and 1%. In this respect patients undergoing carotid endarterectomy are no different from the rest of the population. The suggestion has been made that patients with arteriosclerosis are more likely to have larger intracranial aneurysms than the normal population (Kendall, 1984). The diseased partially obstructed carotid arteries may well have been protecting them from an earlier intracranial or subarachnoid haemorrhage caused by rupture of the aneurysm. It is important, therefore, when asked to anaesthetize a patient for carotid angiography for the assessment of the severity of the carotid artery disease, to bear this in mind and not to use halothane, even though the investigation is to be concentrated on the diseased carotid artery.

In contrast the blood gases act directly on the cerebral capillaries, although Brown and his co-workers (1985) have suggested that it is the oxygen content of the arterial blood that is the more significant. The effect of a high carbon dioxide tension or a low oxygen tension is to dilate the cerebral capillaries. The dominant gas acting on the cerebral vessels for cerebral vasodilatation is carbon dioxide. Conversely, a low carbon dioxide tension or a high oxygen tension cause the cerebral capillaries to be constricted. The dominant gas for capillary constriction is oxygen, although this may be a reflection on the ease by which it is possible to produce high arterial oxygen tensions, particularly in normal subjects.

The changes in cerebral blood flow that follow variation in blood gas tension are transient. Like the cerebral blood flow with chronic changes in arterial blood pressure there is a slow adaptation. This is best seen in climbers adapting to low oxygen tensions when at high altitudes (Severinghaus, 1966), but is also seen when there is chronic carbon dioxide retention. Eventually the degree of capillary vasodilatation re-equilibrates with the new blood gas tension levels and normal cerebral perfusion is restored. If the partial pressure of carbon dioxide is then abruptly lowered to more customary levels, there is marked cerebral vasoconstriction, leading to partial failure of cerebral function, and if sustained for several days, may lead to a depopulation of neurones, i.e. neuronal death. Whilst this has obvious applications in the care of patients with severe chronic respiratory failure, it has, in addition, an application in the care of patients undergoing carotid artery surgery, where fluctuations in capillary run-off have an important bearing on the so-called 'steal' syndrome (Symon, 1969; Pistolese et al., 1971).

The cerebral circulation may be likened to an electrical network of a set of resistors operating in parallel. If one resistor should 'dilate', i.e. its resistance value lessen, more current will flow through it and less current will flow through the other resistors. In normal healthy subjects the vessels act in concert and the ratio of vascular resistances in different parts of the brain is more or less constant, subject only to small variations to meet local metabolic demand. The latter, too, is also reasonably constant as the bulk of the brain's oxygen utilization is to meet the demands for basic cell maintenance rather than is determined by the extent of the local neuronal activity. Oxygen consumption and cerebral blood flow through the cerebral cortex vary little whether the subject is awake and undertaking intense mental activity or is asleep (Ganong, 1982).

In severe cerebral atherosclerosis the situation may be quite different, depending upon the number, location and distribution of the atheromatous plaques. The pulsatile pressure wave in the artery distal to an atheromatous plaque may be dampened and this can increase the risk of an intravascular thrombosis in that for the same mean arterial pressure platelet adhesion to the walls of the vessel is less in pulsatile flow than in steady flow (Sakariassen et al., 1980). Distal to the atheromatous plaque the mean arterial pressure will be low. Optimum flow is dependent both upon pulsatility and mean pressure and so distal to the plaque flow is significantly lowered. Another effect also comes into play in the atheromatous patient. Normally viscosity is of negligible significance when considering flow. Viscous drag occurs principally at the arterioles, where flow is orificial. (Flow through an orifice is determined both by the viscosity and density, or specific gravity, of the moving fluid. Although density is the dominant factor when considering gases flowing through orifices, such as a stenosed trachea, yet when considering the circulation there is little margin for changing the specific gravity of blood so that the specific gravity can be considered as constant. There is a much greater margin for the anaesthetist to change the viscosity of the blood, and so the flow, through any stenosed orifice.) Distal to the arteriole and as a result of the axial streaming, the viscosity of the blood is that of plasma. With a large number of atheromatous plaques there are many more orifices, hence the viscosity can have a significant effect on cerebral blood flow (McHenry et al., 1974). The local auto-regulatory control mechanisms may well be working at their limit in an attempt to preserve the flow. The situation is then like two electrical resistors in series with each other. The resistance is the arithmetical sum of the resistance offered by each of the two resistors. If the atheromatous plaque is the major resistance to flow, reducing the value of the distal resistance by localized vasodilatation will do little to augment flow. If the resistance to flow offered by the atheromatous plaque is sufficiently large, flow may be reduced to a critical level, just enough to maintain cellular viability. Even more important, flow must be just enough to prevent stagnation and local clot formation that the lack of pulsatility favours. This area of the brain is then vulnerable to any one of a number of factors:

1. Driving pressure too low—due to systemic hypotension.
2. Capillary run-off resistance too high—capillary vasoconstriction due to over-ventilation lowering the carbon dioxide tension excessively or raising the oxygen tension excessively.
3. Flow diverted to other areas of lesser resistance because of cerebral vasodilatation. This, in turn, could be because the carbon dioxide tension is too high, or the patient is receiving a drug which relaxes smooth muscle and which is lowering arteriole motor tone. This is the 'steal' syndrome (Symon, 1969).

It follows that if the blood supply to any portion of the brain is precarious, that portion of the brain is likely to be significantly adversely affected by both hypocapnia and hypercapnia. These latter terms are both relative. If there is chronic carbon dioxide retention, the capillaries will have adapted to the higher Paco_2 levels. Any reduction of the Paco_2 to customary normal levels will produce the same response as if there was some hypocapnia. It then follows that the optimum Paco_2 level in a patient with cerebral atherosclerosis is the patient's own resting Paco_2.

There is one other aspect of physiology which can have clinical implications in carotid artery surgery. At the bifurcation of the common carotid artery lie the carotid sinus and carotid body. In normal health these sensors respond to changes in systemic blood pressure and to changes in the arterial blood gas tensions. If the carotid artery wall is diseased by atheromatous plaques at its bifurcation, these sensors cease functioning and are often destroyed in the disease process. Their pressure sensing function is taken over by similar sensors distributed across the body—thus at every major arterial bifurcation and in the aortic arch there are stretch receptors which respond to changes in intraluminal tension produced by the arterial pressure wave, whilst in the brain stem and lateral recesses of the fourth ventricle there are chemoreceptors that respond to changes in blood gas tensions. As a result, the surgeon can usually disrupt the carotid sinus with a fair amount of impunity or by-pass the carotid sinus receptors with a plastic tube as when using a carotid artery by-pass shunt. When this is done, it is rare to see any changes in circulatory haemodynamics. This may not be the case when anaesthetizing a patient undergoing excision of a glomus tumour in the neck.

CLINICAL REQUIREMENTS

Central to carotid artery surgery is the maintenance of normal cerebral perfusion. As has been described, anaesthesia can materially disturb cerebral perfusion in addition to any disturbance produced by the surgeon when the carotid artery is clamped. During general anaesthesia unless there is continuous EEG monitoring one has to infer the adequacy of cerebral perfusion from measuring the stump pressure, that is, the pressure in the distal part of the carotid artery after the surgeon has applied the arterial clamp.

This has led some surgeons to undertake this form of surgery under local anaesthesia, using the patient's level of consciousness as a monitor for cerebral function and so cerebral perfusion, and to help decide whether or not a temporary shunt is necessary during the surgery. Many successful carotid endartectomies have been performed in this way, but the patient has to be very robust emotionally to withstand this—particularly if the patient is aware that he may develop a cerebral infarction or 'stroke' at any time during the procedure. Other surgeons take a different view and prefer general anaesthesia, partly on humanitarian grounds and, partly, to remove the distraction of dealing with perhaps an anxious patient at what could be a critical phase of the operation as well as giving them greater freedom to deal with the surgery or any potential technical problem which may arise during the surgery. In addition, if the patient is anaesthetized and is being artificially ventilated, there is less risk of an unexpected air embolus because of the slight increase in mean intrathoracic pressure, and so central venous pressure, which is a consequence of artificial ventilation.

If general anaesthesia is desired the requirements are straightfor-ward. These are—

1. A high blood pressure and cardiac output
2. Minimum disturbance of cerebral haemodynamics
3. A certain amount of analgesia, although the production of painful stimuli during the operation is not a particular problem
4. A still motionless patient
5. A slightly raised central venous pressure to minimize the risk of air embolism.

The last problem can arise from inadvertent cutting of large veins, particularly the anastomotic venous links between the anterior and external jugular veins. The central venous pressure should not be so high as to cause venous distension within the surgical field.

All these requirements can be met with a relaxant, narcotic, nitrous oxide and artificial ventilation technique combined with a head-up tilt. The degree of head-up tilt is adjusted until the visible veins in the neck collapse at just above the clavicle. At this level there is a slight positive pressure in the veins at the thoracic inlet, which minimizes the risk of air embolism, but the veins in the neck distal to the inlet are above the inlet and their intra-luminal hydrostatic pressure is then zero. Thus a reasonably dry operating field can be obtained.

Pain during carotid artery surgery is not particularly severe, even though the area is well endowed with sensory nerves. This is presumably a direct consequence of the neck's mobility. In contrast to, say, the peritoneum and its sensitivity to stretching and retraction, in the neck all the tissues can be stretched and retracted without producing a lot of pain. The level of analgesia required, although light, is beyond that produced by nitrous oxide alone. Reinforcing the analgesia by hypocapnia, produced by artificial hyperventilation, is not advisable for two reasons (a) the hypocapnia can produce very adverse effects of cerebral blood flow in these patients and (b) the excess ventilation will further raise the intrathoracic pressure and cause unnecessary venous back bleeding within the surgical field. Supplementing the analgesia with a volatile inhalational agent such as halothane runs the risk of the 'steal' syndrome. This risk is less with enflurane at concentrations of 0·5% and yet this concentration contributes enough additional analgesia to be useful. At higher concentrations of enflurane there is a real risk of hypotension and alterations in cerebral haemodynamics. This leaves either the use of narcotics or the combination of general anaesthesia and local anaes-thesia. The local anaesthesia can then be either by cervical epidural block, which has its aficionados, but carries with it all the risks of this particular type of block up to and including cervical cord injury, or by local infiltration. The local infiltration technique must also include good surface anaesthesia to the larynx and trachea to block autonomic reflexes induced by the surgeon moving the head with an endotracheal tube in situ (as must happen at some time during the operation even if only at the towelling and draping-up stage). With the patient obviously asleep and being ventilated, few surgeons would consider the additional complication of administering widespread local infiltration anaesthesia as being worth while.

Narcotic supplementation is then the residual choice. The narcotic can be given either intravenously or intrathecally by lumbar puncture. Intravenous narcotics have the advantage of a very rapid onset, particularly if either phenoperidine or fentanyl is used. However, the duration of analgesia is not long and postoperatively the patient has a fair degree of distress which may not be fully relieved by routine postoperative analgesics. Intrusive postoperative pain can be subdued by intramuscular opiates, but the patient is left with a dull aching wound, marked neck stiffness and inhibition of a fully effective swallowing and laryngeal closure reflex. Laryngeal incompetence remains for some hours with the risk of aspiration atelectasis (Tomlin et al., 1965). Intrathecal opiates provide a greater degree of and a more prolonged analgesia but are slower in onset. With the patient in a 15–20° head-up tilt it takes approximately 15 min before intrathecal morphine blocks the change in heart rate produced by opening the self-retaining retractors in the neck wound. Postoperatively, following intrathecal morphine given at the induction of anaesthesia for carotid artery surgery, the patient appears and behaves as though he had not had an operation. In particular, head and neck movements are completely free with no trace of spasm of either the sternomastoid or the strap muscles—a degree of free movement which some surgeons view with somewhat guarded apprehension. Swallowing, whether of saliva, secretions or oral fluids, is totally unhindered.

A still motionless patient can be achieved by the use of any of the currently available muscle relaxants. In making a choice of relaxant the only important clinical consideration is that there should be as little disturbance of circulatory haemodynamics as possible. Tubocurarine does have some ganglionic blocking effect and this is enhanced with the head-up tilt. The net result is a fall in blood pressure and venous pooling in the dependent part of the body. Although the hypotensive effect can be offset with the use of an adrenergic alpha-stimulating agent, the venous pooling, reduced venous return and therefore the lowered cardiac output are not so responsive. On the other hand, pancuronium appears to potentiate anything likely to stimulate a hypertensive response, including sharp pain. This effect appears to persist into the postoperative period. The pharmacological basis for this is somewhat obscure. Apart from their effects on the circulation, there is little to choose between the different relaxants and so the choice becomes a matter of clinical preference and familiarity.

CLINICAL TECHNIQUE

Preparation and premedication

Patients undergoing reconstructive carotid surgery are usually mature patients with often surprisingly little underlying acute anxiety, although the latter will vary with local conditions. Premedication is not an important component of the anaesthetic technique and it is the author's practice not to give any premedication unless there is a positive indication from the patient. Cigarette smoking, if not already abandoned, should be interdicted for at least 24 hours before anaesthesia in order to minimize any extubation difficulties at the end of the anaesthetic. There is a good case for stopping smoking for 48 hours before anaesthesia. It takes this time before elimination is completed of the deleterious effects on oxygen transport which is the result of the carbon monoxide–haemoglobin complex which cigarette smoking produces (Davies et al., 1979). Otherwise, the preparation and evaluation are the same as for any other major vascular operation.

Induction

The choice of induction agent is wide and will depend upon the anaesthetist's preference, subject to the usual possible pharmacological idiosyncrasies or drug sensitivities. The patients with arterial disease frequently have very slow arm–brain circulation times, double or even treble that of younger, fitter patients, so that a modest degree of care is necessary to avoid giving a relative over-dose of induction agent.

Intubation

There are no undue difficulties with intubation which are specific to patients undergoing carotid artery surgery, although these patients are elderly and often have a certain amount of cervical spondylosis. As a consequence some care is necessary when extending the head. However, the major problem occurs during the draping of the head and neck when the head will be moved and this will cause some movement of the endotracheal tube within the trachea, which will cause an outburst of autonomic activity. To avoid this type of stimulation disturbing the patient it is a useful precaution to apply surface anaesthesia with a local anaesthetic spray immediately prior to intubation. Towards the end of the operation the surgeon is likely to request some head flexion whilst he rejoins any muscles he has divided. If a soft rubber endotracheal tube has been used, there is a slight risk that the tube may then kink. As the mouth is usually tightly covered with drapes, access in order to unkink the tube may be difficult. It is a prudent precaution, therefore, to use a tube which is unlikely to kink, such as a reinforced latex tube, or a synthetic tube such as a Portex tube. Since the tube will be led backwards over the eyes and the top of the head and subsequently be covered by drapes, the eyes should be well protected against accidental abrasions.

Infusion lines

It is a fundamental axiom of arterial surgery that there could be a major and very rapid haemorrhage at any time either due to a ligature or clamp slipping or due to the artery tearing. In this one respect arterial surgery and arterial surgeons are not to be trusted. During carotid artery surgery, although the vessels are easily visible and surgical access not a problem so that blood loss is likely to be minimal, yet it is important to have a drip established that is capable, if necessary, of coping with a rapid blood transfusion.

Monitoring

The most important single part of monitoring in carotid artery surgery is the arterial blood pressure. This must be continuously monitored throughout the whole operation. For optimum patient care periodic sampling whether by auscultation or oscillotonometry, automatic or otherwise, is not sufficient. There is no substitute for an invasive method, such as radial artery cannulation and direct recording or display on an oscilloscope. The system has the additional advantage of being available for the measurement of the distal stump pressure during the period of carotid occlusion.

At some stage the surgeon will want to measure the stump pressure. This is best done by an additional monitoring line to the transducer which is being used to measure the systemic arterial pressure. Oscilloscopic display of a good pulsatile pressure wave or a mean stump pressure greater than 80 mmHg indicates that a temporary intracarotid shunt is unnecessary.

If a transducer is not available, a simple anaeroid manometer hydraulically coupled to the radial artery cannula is an inexpensive alternative. In this system a narrow bore, stiff, sterile plastic tube is connected to the radial artery cannula via a three-way stopcock at the wrist. The other end of the tube is joined via another three-way stopcock to the anaeroid manometer. The tubing is then filled, up to the level of the distal stopcock, with sterile saline to which a little heparin has been added. After purging all the bubbles from the tubing, the anaeroid manometer is suspended above the tubing and all taps are then opened to it. The needle of the anaeroid manometer will then swing with each heart beat. The pressure signal is slightly damped, due to the compressible volume of air within the actual chamber of the anaeroid manometer (this chamber is deliberately left full of air because of the risk of corrosion, as well as the difficulties of sterilization). Therefore the pressure signal is not quite as accurate as a complete electromanometric transducer system, yet it is as accurate as any indirect method of measuring the blood pressure. It also has the advantage of showing the blood pressure from every heart beat. Due to the compressible volume of air within the anaeroid chamber a small quantity of blood pulsates in and out of the proximal centimetre of the manometer line, and this is the reason for the added heparin. All purgings and wash-outs of the tubing should be through the stopcock which is by the wrist—in this way accidental bacteriological contamination will be avoided.

There are three other items of monitoring equipment which provide useful practical information. These are: (a) equipment for end tidal carbon dioxide measurement, which is invaluable in helping maintain an optimum P_{CO_2} level, (b) an ECG monitor, these patients have arterial disease and it must be assumed that there is at least some subclinical coronary artery disease and therefore arrhythmias are likely, and (c) some method of sensing the brain's electrical activity. A conventional diagnostic EEG machine with multi-channel leads and continuous surveillance by an expert electroencephalographist is ideal. Small variations in cerebral perfusion will be readily detected and the appropriate corrections made to the anaesthetic or surgical technique. A skilful expert can even distinguish between the anaesthetic styles of different anaesthetists anaesthetizing different patients for carotid endarterectomy—double blind! The alternative is a cerebral function monitor. A recent improvement has been the development of a frequency-amplitude wave analyser. This device analyses trains of EEG waves for both frequency and amplitude. If the signals for frequency and amplitude converge, this means periods of electrical silence—a sign of either too deep an anaesthetic or a depressed brain. Lesser degrees of cerebral dysfunction produce delta waves —of large amplitude but low frequency. The analyser will show this very clearly.

An alternative to sensing the brain's electrical activity is to measure continuously the conjunctival oxygen tension by means of a surface oxygen electrode. The lateral parts of the conjunctiva, sclera and cornea are supplied by branches of the ophthalmic artery, itself a division of the internal carotid artery. There is a small anastomosis with the facial artery at the medial corner of the eye but the main anastomoses are through the circle of Willis. If at the time of clamping the carotid artery the blood supply from the circle of Willis is inadequate then the ipsilateral brain and eye will become hypoxic. This will be reflected in the oxygen tension of the conjunctiva. Thus, monitoring consists of inserting a small surface oxygen electrode into the lateral part of the conjuctival sac immediately after the induction of anaesthesia and then continuously measuring the conjunctival oxygen tension. If the oxygen tension level should fall after clamping the carotid this is an indication of inadequate oxygenation and the need for the surgeon to insert a temporary bypass shunt into the internal carotid artery. It should be emphasized that the conjunctival oxygen tension is a reflection of brain-tissue oxygenation and not the arterial oxygen tension.

Maintenance

This is best achieved with a nitrous oxide–relaxant technique supplemented with narcotics and a trace of enflurane, for reasons previously discussed in this chapter. The intrathoracic pressure can be adjusted by suitable manipulation of the negative phase controls so that the veins are just visible at the level of the clavicle with a head-up tilt. This corresponds to a mean intrathoracic pressure of approximately $3 \, \text{cmH}_2\text{O}$. This combination achieves total lack of awareness with a very light plane of anaesthesia. Alternative methods have been used but they carry with them a greater likelihood of a disturbance in cerebral haemodynamics, such as lowering the level of activity of the vasomotor centre or episodes of awareness during the anaesthetic.

Reversal and recovery

Reversal of the relaxant at the end of anaesthesia poses no particular problems, although the act of extubation can have a great arousal effect and stimulate a burst of severe hypertension. It is perhaps better to extubate as soon as the reversal agents take effect and before discontinuing the trace concentration of inhalational agent. This will mitigate against some of the excessive hypertension.

POSTOPERATIVE PROBLEMS

Apart from the complications that are common to all anaesthesia and surgery—infection, pulmonary problems, deep vein thrombosis etc.—there are certain problems that are more specific to this form of vascular surgery.

1. Haemorrhage

Like all forms of arterial surgery haemorrhage from the arteriotomy is a definite risk. Unless the haematoma can escape, the risk is of displacement, kinking or possible compression of the larynx—in this it is not unlike the problem of haemorrhage following thyroid surgery. Emergency relief of the compression is essential as the compression may result in carotid artery occlusion with the risk of some cerebral infarction.

2. Thrombosis of the artery

This is a rare but severe problem. It frequently means some permanent cerebral damage. Surgical intervention to remove the clot is rarely of benefit. High-dose steroids might minimize the amount of cerebral damage, but the evidence that they confer any benefit is very doubtful.

3. Hypertension

The major postoperative problem is the hypertension that follows major arterial surgery. This lasts only 2–3 hours but can put a very severe mechanical stress on the suture lines. The aetiology is obscure but the level of hypertension can be severe, with peak systolic pressures as high as 300 mmHg. Fortunately, the duration per heart beat of the pulse of very high pressure is usually very brief. In fact, so brief that the more conventional auscultatory methods of measuring the blood pressure fail to detect it. If there is any doubt about the hypertension, then hypotensive agents should be used. Continuous infusion systems are better as they can be rapidly discontinued when the hypertensive phase ceases. Trimetaphan or sodium nitroprusside or trinitrate can be used. Other methods include heavy sedation with narcotics or with alpha-blocking agents such as chlorpromazine. If the surgery has been successful in improving overall cerebral blood flow, there should be little risk that the resulting vasodilatation will precipitate a 'steal' syndrome.

4. Intracranial aneurysm

One rare but important complication of this hypertension is a rupture of a small intracranial aneurysm. It is important to establish, as soon as the patient is awake and can cooperate, that the patient can freely move all four limbs. This enables the correct diagnosis to be made in the event of any subsequent hemiplegia with a good pulsating carotid artery, otherwise it may be attributed to an intra-operative mishap, or may precipitate an unnecessary re-exploration of the neck.

172   ANAESTHESIA FOR VASCULAR SURGERY

5. Vagal stimulation

Another, but very rare and important, complication of carotid artery surgery is a haematoma within the carotid sheath stretching and so stimulating the vagus nerve. This will cause a marked bradycardia, hypotension and clouding of consciousness. A useful diagnostic test is to give 0·5–0·6 mg atropine intravenously. If this restores the pulse rate and blood pressure to normal and causes an improvement in the level of consciousness, only for it all to relapse when the atropine wears off, the diagnosis is obvious. It is then up to the surgical team to decide whether to remove the haematoma or not.

6. Upper airway obstruction

A quite different complication following carotid artery surgery is acute upper airway obstruction, due to either laryngeal nerve palsy or laryngeal oedema. It is very rare after simple carotid endarterectomy but is a definite risk if the surgery is more extensive, e.g. removing a glomus tumour or removing a carotid artery aneurysm. Treatment of either is by endotracheal intubation, which may need to be maintained for several days. If the nerve palsy is late in onset then it is most likely to be due to nerve oedema and the outlook is correspondingly more favourable.

REFERENCES

Brown M. M., Wade P. P. H. and Marshall J. (1985) Fundamental importance of arterial oxygen content in the regulation of cerebral blood flow in man. *Brain* **108**, 81

Davies J. M., Latto I. P., Jones J. G. et al. (1979) Effects of stopping smoking for 48 hours on oxygen availability from the blood. *Br. Med. J.* **2**, 355

Eastcott H. H. G., Pickering G. W. and Rob C. G. (1954) Reconstruction of the internal carotid artery in a patient with intermittent attacks of hemiplegia. *Lancet* **ii**, 994

Ganong W. F. (1983) Regulation of cerebral circulation. In: *Review of Medical Physiology*, 11th edn. p. 495. Lange Medical Publications, California

Harper A. M. (1966) Autoregulation of cerebral blood flow: Influence of the arterial blood pressure on the blood flow through the cerebral cortex. *J. Neurol. Neurosurg. Psychiatry* **29**, 398

Heistad D. D. and Kontos H. A. (1983) The cerebral circulation. In: *Handbook of Physiology: Cardiovascular System*, vol. 3., p. 1145. Am. Physiol. Soc., Bethesda, Maryland

Iwayama T., Furness J. B. and Burnstock G. (1970) Dual adrenergic and cholinergic innervation of the cerebral arteries in the rat. *Circ. Res.* **26**, 635

Keele C. A., Neil E. and Joels N. (1982) The cerebral circulation. In: *Samson Wright's Applied Physiology*. 13th edn., p. 138. Oxford University Press, Oxford

Kendall B. (1984) Angiography of the head. Evidence of a common factor in the aetiology of larger intracranial aneurysms and atherosclerosis. In: *Textbook of Radiological Diagnosis*, 5th edn., p. 200. Editor: Boulay G. H. D. Roy. Coll. Radiol. Lewis, London

Landau W. M. (1955) The local circulation in the living brain. *Trans. Am. Neurol. Assoc.* **80**, 125

McDowell G. (1965) The effects of anaesthetics on cerebral blood flow and cerebral metabolism. *Br. J. Anaesth.* **37**: 236

McDowell G. (1970). In: *The Cerebral Circulation*. Little Brown, Boston

McHenry L. C., West J. W., Cooper E. S. et al. (1974) Cerebral autoregulation in man. *Stroke* **5**, 695

O'Brien M. D. (1967) Cerebral cortex perfusion rates in migraine. *Lancet* **i**, 1036

Pistolese G. R., Citone G., Faragloia V. et al. (1971) The effects of hypercapnia on cerebral blood flow during clamping of the carotid arteries in the surgical management of cerebrovascular insufficiency. *Neurol. Minneap.* **21**, 95

Sakariassen K. S., Bolhuis P. A. and Sixma J. J. (1980) Platelet adherence to the subendothelium of human arteries in pulsatile and steady flow. *Thrombosis Res.* **415**, 547

Selkoe D. J. and Myers R. E. (1979) Neurological and cardiovascular effects of hypotension in the monkey. *Stroke* **10**, 147

Severinghaus J. W. (1966) Cerebral blood flow at high altitudes. *Circ. Res.* **19**, 274

Sokoloff L. and Kety S. S. (1960) Regulation of the cerebral circulation. *Physiol. Rev.* **40**, Suppl. 4

Stephenson H. E. (1974) Cerebral anoxia and neurologic sequelae. In: *Cardiac Arrest and Resuscitation*, 4th edn., p. 455. Mosby, London

Symon L. (1969) The concept of intracerebral steal. *Int. Anesthesiol. Clin.* **7**, 597

Tomlin P. J., Howarth F. H. and Robinson J. S. (1965) Postoperative atelectasis and laryngeal incompetence. *Lancet* **i**, 1462

Tomlin P. J., Martin J. W. and Honisberger L. (1981) Brain Death: A retrospective survey. *Lancet* **i**, 378

Warren J. V. (1974) Physiology of the giraffe. *Scient. Am.* **231**, 5 : 96

CHAPTER 7

Other Vascular Operations

Apart from those discussed earlier in this book, there are a number of other operations undertaken by vascular surgeons—some rare, some common—which pose problems for the anaesthetist. Most of these problems can be managed by the judicious application of the general principles described earlier in this book; some though require particular consideration. These operations are:

> Cervical sympathectomy
> Axillo-femoral by-pass graft surgery
> Thoraco-abdominal aortic surgery
> Subdiaphragmatic suprarenal aneurysms
> Pulmonary embolectomy
> Dissecting aneurysms

CERVICAL SYMPATHECTOMY

The clinical origin of patients requiring cervical sympathectomy has a much wider range than the usual run of patients presenting for vascular surgery. They range from the young, fit, healthy patient with socially inhibiting hyperhydrosis of the hand, include patients with severe post-traumatic causalgia and patients with Raynaud's disease, to patients with phantom limb pain following forequarter amputation for upper limb cancer. The surgical approach to cervical sympathectomy is very different for different surgeons and this materially affects the anaesthetic management. Broadly, the surgical approach is either through the posterior triangle of the neck or an axillary transthoracic approach.

The cervical approach

In this approach the surgeon aims to reach the stellate ganglion and its branches via the neck. The patient will therefore be draped in a manner similar to that used for thyroid operations so that an endotracheal tube will be necessary to ensure full patency of the airways.

During the operation there are a number of technical hazards that the surgeon must overcome and about which the anaesthetist must be aware in case the surgeon has difficulties. Foremost of these is the unintentional opening of the pleura. The sympathetic nerves lies immediately adjacent to Simpson's fascia, a layer of fascia that forms the roof of the thoracic cavity lying within the arch of the first rib. If this fascia is opened, the result is a pneumothorax. More important is the fact that if the anaesthetic technique which has been used up to that point is one involving spontaneous respiration, the anaesthetist must convert the anaesthetic technique immediately to one of controlled ventilation, if major lung collapse is to be avoided. There are advocates for the spontaneous respiration technique, the justification being that during spontaneous respiration the venous pressure within the neck will be lower than that occurring during controlled respiration. This, therefore, gives improved surgical conditions and shortens the operating and anaesthetic time. Furthermore, some surgeons are extremely adept at this operation, completing it within 10–15 min which is inconvenient when a non-depolarizing relaxant has been used, although the recent introduction of atracurium has alleviated this problem.

Another surgical hazard is the unintentional division of a major lymphatic channel, the thoracic duct on the left or its homologue on the right. Although the long-term consequences of this are of no major significance (any chilous fistula usually settles eventually), the intra-operative problems of an obscured surgical field can be of considerable nuisance value and commonly mean a somewhat protracted operation and anaesthetic, which can be a disadvantage if the short-acting muscle relaxant atracurium is being used.

The third surgical problem that the surgeon faces is haemorrhage. In the transcervical sympathectomy the surgeon has to find his way between a number of major vessels such as the transcervical and suprascapular vessels. He also passes close to the vertebral vessels and the subclavian vessels. Any of these vessels can be accidentally damaged, but the most difficult to deal with is the damaged subclavian vein. Unlike most veins the subclavian vein does not collapse when cut. It is held open by various sheets of fascia. Surgical access to a damaged subclavian vein from above can be technically particularly difficult so that blood loss of a litre or more can result. Worse is if the pleura has been opened. Then much of the blood may leak into the chest and form a large concealed haemorrhage. Fortunately this complication is very rare yet, nevertheless, it is one for which the anaesthetist must be prepared. If the vein has been opened, it is prudent to try to maintain a small positive intrathoracic pressure to minimize the risk of an air embolism.

Although there are those anaesthetists who favour spontaneous respiration via an endotracheal tube for patients undergoing supraclavicular cervical sympathectomy, with the option of changing to controlled ventilation if the occasion warrants it, this is by no means universal. Owing to the fact that this particular anaesthetic technique requires the inhalation of an anaesthetic vapour of high concentration (in order to tolerate the presence of the endotracheal tube in the trachea), it is inappropriate for patients with peripheral vascular disease because of the risk of hypotension. This method of anaesthesia is best reserved for younger patients such as those undergoing cervical sympathectomy for hyperhydrosis. Even then the controlled ventilation technique allows for a faster recovery period. If the technique of spontaneous ventilation is chosen, an important component of the technique is a thorough spraying of the vocal cords prior to intubation. This tends to minimize the concentration of volatile agent which needs to be given.

The general principles of anaesthetic management for a transcervical sympathectomy in the vascular patient involve intubation, controlled ventilation and venous cannulation, using a large venous cannula so that a large blood transfusion can be given rapidly should the occasion warrant. The choice of anaesthetic agents to achieve these objectives will depend upon the patient's background medical condition and the anaesthetist's preference and familiarity with particular anaesthetic agents.

The patient is positioned with a head-up tilt sufficient to collapse the neck veins to the level of the clavicle. Monitoring should be by indirect means, using an electrocardiograph and some form of sphygmomanometer or oscillotonometer—preferably an automated electronic one. Arterial cannulation for the direct measurement of the arterial blood pressure is unnecessary and is specifically contraindicated in those patients suffering from Raynaud's disease. If during the operation the pleura has been inadvertently opened, the lungs should be fully re-expanded to drive out any pneumothorax as the surgeon closes the various fascial layers. If this complication has arisen during surgery, then immediately postoperatively the patient should have a chest radiograph taken sitting up to ensure that there is no concealed haemothorax.

The transthoracic approach

In this approach the surgeon enters the chest via the axilla to reach the stellate ganglion and the second thoracic ganglion. (Sometimes this is fused with the stellate ganglion; in other patients it is a discrete entity.) It is principally the branches of the latter that form most of the sympathetic nerve supply to the upper limb. The clinical advantages of this approach are that there is very much less risk of damaging the sympathetic nerve supply to the head and face, so that a Horner's syndrome is much less likely. There is considerably less risk of damaging a major blood vessel or lymphatic vessel. Once inside the chest vision and surgical access to the upper sympathetic chain are very easy, although achieving optimal illumination is occasionally difficult and may require some lung retraction.

From the anaesthetist's viewpoint the operation must be regarded as a full thoracic operation requiring total control of the ventilation and lung volumes. The patient is positioned on his side with the affected side uppermost. The uppermost arm is held high and supported on the frame of the anaesthetist's screen in order to expose the axilla fully. This means that the sphygmomanometer cuff should be placed upon the dependent arm. A cuffed double-lumen endo-bronchial tube is unnecessary; a simple endotracheal tube will suffice providing that the tidal volumes and inflationary pressures are not too high. When the chest is opened, the exposed lung will collapse slightly but either a lung retractor or a large moist swab will be all that is necessary to compress it further in order to improve surgical access to the sympathetic chain. At the time of chest closure the lungs will need re-expanding to dispel any air from the pleural cavity. As the surgeon has not, or should not have, damaged the visceral pleura, there should be no risk of pneumothorax and provided that haemo-stasis is sound there is no need for any chest drains. Again, post-operatively a sitting chest radiograph is the best for detecting any residual pneumothorax or haemothorax.

Many of the patients presenting for transthoracic cervical sympath-ectomy have stable circulatory systems and can easily withstand the transient changes in haemodynamics caused by re-expanding the lungs. However, if there is widespread atherosclerotic disease, some care is necessary so that neither too high nor too sudden an increased intrathoracic pressure is produced when re-expanding the lungs, as either of these can produce a sharp fall in venous return, cardiac output and hypotension which may not recover quite so quickly as it does in the more circulatory robust patients.

Monitoring during anaesthesia for a transthoracic cervical sym-pathectomy is the same as when the cervical approach is used.

AXILLO-FEMORAL BY-PASS GRAFT SURGERY

In this operation the surgeon aims to insert a vascular prosthesis joining the axillary or subclavian artery to the ipsilateral femoral or external iliac artery. Often there is an associated femoral–femoral cross-over graft to be performed as well. The vascular grafts are all placed subcutaneously down the whole length of the anterolateral aspect of the trunk and across the anterior abdominal wall just above the symphysis pubis.

This operation generates four matters that are of particular concern to the anaesthetist:

1. Ischaemic disease

Patients undergoing this operation usually have very severe and widespread degenerative vascular disease, such that the aorta has become too diseased for any useful operation. Therefore, atheromatous deposits are more than usually likely to be widespread through many of the major arteries, including the coronary and the cerebral arteries. Thus, more than most patients undergoing vascular surgery, these patients are more vulnerable to the consequences of hypotension. Yet in these patients a burst of hypotension is more likely. As a consequence of their widespread degenerative disease, there is very considerable loss of elastic tissue in the medial layer of the major arteries (Walter and Israel, 1979). Perfusion, therefore, relies critically on a very hard working heart so that each stroke volume is delivered at high velocity and high pressure in order to maintain normal perfusion rates. With so much degeneration of elastic tissue in the aorta, the elastic recoil is very little and diastolic flow is reduced to a bare minimum. As a direct consequence there must be the minimum disturbance of systolic ejection. These hearts are particularly sensitive to any trace of myocardial depressant agent so that, during anaesthesia, hypotension is much more likely to occur should any such agent be given, even if the dose is very small. Furthermore, these hearts are very slow to recover from hypotension. As a group among all patients presenting for arterial surgery, the patients requiring axillo-femoral by-pass surgery rank among the highest as being the most brittle of hypertensive patients, and their widespread atheroma makes them particularly vulnerable to the hypotension precipitating ischaemia and thrombosis. Apart from myocardial depression, there are two other important sources of hypotension—blood loss and pain. In these patients, again more often than in other groups of patients undergoing vascular surgery, the response to pain is a vagal response with a marked bradycardia, a reduced cardiac output and hypotension.

2. The subcutaneous tunnelling

This is usually performed by blunt dissection, often by thrusting blind under the skin a large obturator tube with the diameter of a sigmoidoscope. This particular phase of the operation is very painful so that good quality analgesia is essential if reflex hypotension is to be avoided.

3. The vascular prosthesis

This is a long one and is particularly liable to clotting in the first half-hour or so of use, until platelet deposition has helped form a smooth lining. Other factors leading to clotting within the graft are kinking of the graft and a poor run-off opposing forward flow and reducing the velocity of flow. Once the run-off to both legs is established, clot formation within the graft is less of a problem. The anaesthetist's role in preventing clot formation within the graft is to ensure that the velocity of blood flow does not falter. It is essential to prevent any hypotension occurring in the early stages after the circulation to the legs has been re-established.

4. Monitoring

The operation is usually performed on the right side of the body. This means that the arterial blood supply to the right arm will be interrupted by the surgeon. It is important, therefore, that the arterial line which is to be used for monitoring the arterial pressure be inserted into the left radial artery. If, for any reason, such as severe atheromatous deposits in the right subclavian or axillary artery, the surgeon is forced to use the left side, then the right radial artery should be used for monitoring.

Apart from ascertaining from the surgeon which side he will be operating upon prior to starting the anaesthetic, the anaesthetist should review the angiographic films—almost invariably these patients will have had an arch aortogram performed a few days prior to surgery. What the anaesthetist is looking for is the degree, if any, of obstruction to blood flow in the subclavian or axillary artery on the side which is to be used for monitoring. If either of these arteries is obstructed, there will be very extensive collateral anastomoses around the shoulder joint. These anastomoses will ensure that the upper limb is viable, but it does mean that there is a real risk of attenuation and damping of the blood pressure signal sensed from the ipsilateral radial artery. As a consequence, the anaesthetist may gain a false picture of the arterial pressure. Preoperative sphygmomanometry of both arms will confirm any suspected difference.

If there is a difference in blood pressure measured in the two arms and the prospective monitoring arm has the lower pressure, then a useful way of dealing with this problem is to cannulate both radial arteries and join the two pressure lines to a three-way tap, which is then joined to the dome of the pressure transducer. Any difference in blood pressure recorded from the two arms is then added to the value obtained from the monitoring arm. Paired values are then taken frequently, of blood pressure from the two arms, up to the time that the surgeon clamps the subclavian artery. By this time, hopefully, the anaesthetist will have obtained a set of values of the differences in arterial pressure between the two arms over a range of pressures and should have some idea of what level of damped pressure corresponds to the optimal blood pressure. Although this is not an ideal preliminary, the anaesthetist then will be in a better position to compensate for any damping once the subclavian clamp has been applied. It should perhaps be appreciated that patients with arterial disease of the upper half of the body have a slightly greater than normal risk of radial artery problems following radial artery cannulation (Samaan, 1971), although this risk is still very, very small and the advantages of radial artery cannulation significantly outweigh the disadvantages.

An alternative, but technically less satisfactory approach is to cannulate the superficial temporal artery. In these elderly arteriopathic patients the superficial temporal artery is easy to palpate. But it is usually very thick-walled with a narrow lumen and so tortuous in the elderly that threading the arterial cannula well into the artery is often impossible, so that only the cannula tip lies in the artery, vulnerable to any minor external movement of the cannula or the patient's head. Alternatives to the superficial temporal artery are the carotid and the facial arteries. Cannulating the carotid artery just for the purpose of monitoring the blood pressure is unjustified because of the risk of minor emboli to the brain, whilst cannulating the facial artery is technically extremely difficult because of the sharp bend it makes at the only point where it can be palpated, where the artery crosses the lower border of the mandible.

As a last resort, automated electronic sphygmomanometry will provide some indication of the blood pressure and this, coupled with the electrocardiograph and the anaesthetist's experience and knowledge of the drugs which have been used, should at least ensure that dangerous degrees of hypotension are not occurring. This form of monitoring though is less satisfactory and in particular the quality of the information such as that derived from the shape of the arterial pressure wave will not be obtained.

THORACO-ABDOMINAL AORTIC SURGERY

The need for thoraco-abdominal aortic surgery arises from three distinct population groups. The first are the patients with degenerative atherosclerosis, the second are patients with traumatic rupture of the thoracic aorta (usually the result of a road accident), whilst the third group are patients with Marfan's syndrome. Patients with Marfan's syndrome presenting for vascular surgery are usually very much younger than the conventional arteriopathic patient. They do not have widespread atherosclerosis so that compensatory hypertension and high systolic blood velocity are not so much a feature. As a consequence, the majority withstand the vicissitudes of anaesthesia and surgery, hypotension and blood loss considerably better than the average arterial surgery patient. However, a significant number of the

Marfan syndrome patients have associated heart disease. Roberts (1979) in a detailed pathological study found that, at post mortem, half the Marfan syndrome patients had pathological hearts. This commonly was incompetence of the aortic or mitral valve or both. The valve disorders were due to connective tissue damage of either the valve leaflets or the valve ring. Hirst and Gore (1973) in a review of Marfan's syndrome, noted that about one-third of the patients had clinical heart disease. Marfan syndrome patients often have multiple aneurysms, not only of the aorta but frequently of the iliac, femoral and even popliteal arteries.

Traumatic rupture of the descending aorta is often part of a picture of multiple injuries but its clinical management is not dissimilar to that of intrathoracic aneurysms (Turney et al., 1976). Pure intra-thoracic aneurysms below the arch of the aorta are comparatively rare, as there is very little turbulent flow in the intrathoracic descend-ing aorta and turbulence is the major immediate precipitating factor in aneurysm formation. Providing the surgeon inserts a temporary vascular by-pass linking the upper and lower halves of the body, the anaesthetic problems, in the management of a patient undergoing resection of an intrathoracic aneurysm of the descending aorta, are not dissimilar to those arising in the anaesthetic management of a patient with coarctation of the aorta. The principal problem of this type of surgery is occlusion of the spinal arteries, particularly those of the lower thoracic vertebra (Crawford et al., 1978). Infarction of the spinal cord, paraplegia and spinal shock due to loss of the lower part of the sympathetic outflow are sufficiently common to deter most surgeons from resecting such aneurysms (Stoney and Wylie, 1973). Alternative operations such as inducing extensive clot formation in the aneurysm by inserting foreign bodies within the aneurysm cavity (Rob and De Weese, 1979) or splinting the aneurysm to prevent it over-distending have all been and are still being tried. From an anaesthetic viewpoint, these operations present no particular difficul-ties beyond those common to elderly vascular surgery patients undergoing thoracotomy (Dunbar, 1979). It is a wise precaution in these patients not to use intrathecal or epidural analgesics as if there is a spinal artery thrombosis with consequent paraplegia, aetiology may be wrongly attributed, with perhaps unnecessary investigations or even consideration of a laminectomy under the misapprehension that the paraplegia is due to a haematoma within the spinal canal.

SUBDIAPHRAGMATIC SUPRARENAL ANEURYSMS

Subdiaphragmatic suprarenal aneurysms present a formidable chal-lenge both to surgeon and anaesthetist (Crawford et al., 1978). A significant factor in the clinical management is whether the aneurysm involves the coeliac axis and its associated hepatic artery. If so, almost invariably the superior mesenteric artery is also involved. Between the two they take more than a quarter of the cardiac output. The inferior mesenteric artery is less important provided that the superior mesenteric and superior haemorrhoidal arteries are patent as the lower bowel will normally survive on the marginal artery that links the mesenteric cascades, middle colic artery and superior haemorrhoidal artery. Neither the superior mesenteric artery nor the superior haemorrhoidal artery is capable of supplying the whole of the blood supply of the lower bowel by itself.

If the aneurysm involves the coeliac axis, then the blood supply to the liver, small bowel and both kidneys will be interrupted for a period of time during the surgery. At normothermia the healthy liver can withstand total ischaemia for approximately 30 min, the kidneys somewhat longer. Friedman and his co-workers (1954) have shown that following half an hour of total ischaemia, the kidneys will recover with little to no damage. Experimentally, they also found that, even with 2 hours of total ischaemia, there will be renal tubular damage but with an excellent prospect of eventual recovery. In clinical practice the maximum renal ischaemic time in patients undergoing suprarenal aortic surgery is about 90 min (Gore and Hirst, 1973). The major risk from this type of surgery is still spinal cord damage from occlusion of the lumbar arteries. Nevertheless, to avoid significant liver damage the surgeon must complete the key stages of the operation in half an hour or so. In that time the surgeon must clamp the aorta and cut squares out of the aorta which contain the origin of the coeliac axis and superior mesenteric arteries, plus additional squares for the two renal arteries. He then has to perform the upper aortic anastomosis between the aorta and graft, and insert the various squares into the graft to re-establish the blood flow to these vital organs. It is a very considerable technical challenge to the surgeon and so the operation is very rarely performed. Once this vital blood flow is re-established, the lower aortic anastomosis can be completed at leisure.

The anaesthetic problems are also marked. During the period of aortic occlusion the increase in aortic impedance is very substantial as approximately half the cardiac output was going to the subdiaphragmatic organs and this run-off is suddenly obstructed. The arterial pressure rises very rapidly and imposes a considerable strain on the left ventricle. Conversely, at the time of re-establishing hepatic blood flow there is a dramatic fall in aortic impedance and with it a sharp fall in blood pressure, which may require a very rapid blood transfusion to restore normotension. Inevitably, there is some metabolic acidosis arising from the ischaemic liver, although this is often self-correcting. However, it is the mechanical stresses on the left ventricle which form the major cause for concern. These can be ameliorated by the infusion of a short-acting vasodilator agent such as sodium nitroprusside or trinitrate during the period of aortic cross-clamping. The rate of infusion is then titrated against the patient's blood pressure. Critical liaison with the surgeon is essential as the surgeon approaches the stage of releasing the aortic clamp.

If the aneurysm involves only the renal arteries, the situation is slightly less hurried and the changes in aortic impedance are less severe. The major risk is of renal artery thrombosis and kidney infarction, although this risk is lessened by the surgeon injecting a large volume of dilute heparin into the aneurysm, some of which inevitably will flow down the renal arteries. The other hazard is acute tubular necrosis. This not infrequently occurs. With modern renal dialysis techniques this is not the life-threatening condition that it once was. The acute tubular necrosis should recover within 6 weeks, and often recovers earlier than that.

If a normothermic technique of anaesthesia is used for the management of a patient undergoing suprarenal aortic surgery, or renal artery surgery, it is important to give a bolus of diuretic, such as frusemide, immediately after the restoration of renal artery blood flow. This appears to reduce the risk and severity of acute tubular necrosis.

Attempts have been made to minimize these complications and to prolong the ischaemic period by the use of induced hypothermia. These attempts have had little success. The overall results including survival when hypothermia has been used and when normothermia has been used are not significantly different (Crawford and Rubio, 1973). That is to say, the complications and morbidity associated with hypothermia counterbalance the gains obtained from prolonging the ischaemia time.

The problems associated with induced hypothermia for correction of a suprarenal aneurysm are, broadly, twofold: (1) technical and (2) physiological.

1. The technical problems of induced hypothermia

Inevitably the hypothermia is performed by surface cooling in which the patient, complete with all monitoring lines in situ, is immersed in a bath filled with ice-cold water. These patients are frequently very obese. During the surface cooling a considerable temperature gradient develops between the core temperature and the skin with its subcutaneous tissues. This happens with all surface-cooling techniques and is recognized by allowing for an after-drop in body temperature on removing the patient from the cold bath. In the young and frequently slim patient undergoing heart surgery under hypothermia the average size of the after-drop is approximately 2 °C

(Atkinson et al., 1982a). In the obese arteriopathic patient the size of the after-drop is considerably more variable and uncontrollable. It can be as much as 5 °C. The large size of the after-drop in temperature is in part due to the poor peripheral circulation that these patients have so that heat and cold transport across different parts of the body is much less efficient, and as a result there is greater difficulty in the body reaching thermal equilibrium between the very cold subcutaneous fat and the warmer core temperature, and in part due to their large body mass relative to the mass of the central core. Significant gain in ischaemic time is not achieved until the core temperature lies between 32 and 30 °C as the metabolic rate and oxygen demand falls by 8–10% (Maclean and Emslie-Smith, 1977; Atkinson et al., 1982b). A 50% reduction in oxygen demand will not be achieved until the core temperature reaches these levels. Another matter that must also be taken into account is the time taken to achieve hypothermia. In these patients this can be very prolonged.

An after-drop of 4–5 °C would take the core temperature well below the safety level into the region of hypothermically induced ventricular fibrillation (Atkinson et al., 1982c). There is a strong clinical suspicion, although objective proof is almost impossible to obtain, that the temperature threshold at which ventricular fibrillation occurs is higher in the patient with peripheral vascular disease, particularly if that disease involves the coronary circulation.

To reverse the ventricular fibrillation requires cardiac massage, either external or transdiaphragmatic, the application of copious amounts of warm saline into the peritoneal cavity, to rewarm the inferior vena cava and the liver, thereby increasing the liver's metabolic rate and heat production, and the application of electrical defibrillation.

2. The physiological problems of hypothermia

The disorders of physiology that accompany induced hypothermia in the arteriopathic patient relate mainly to the circulatory system. Hypothermia induces a marked bradycardia, a reduction in cardiac output (the cardiac output falls exponentially with the reduction in core temperature; Tomlin et al., 1966), and a reduction in myocardial contractility. There are reductions in the rate of acceleration of blood flow as it is ejected into the aorta, in mean flow velocity as well as peak flow as measured at the proximal part of the ascending aorta, and most significant of all, a marked hypotension. If there are any partially occluded vessels which contain patches of roughened intima, the reduction in flow, pressure and velocity of flow predispose to thrombus formation at these atheromatous plaques, notwithstanding the prolongation of clotting time that hypothermia induces. The end-result is increased morbidity.

Allied to this problem of hypotension are the pharmacological actions of the drug used to promote hypothermia. Chlorpromazine is a powerful dopamine-blocking agent (Pharmaceutical Codex, 1979a) and so can precipitate a marked hypotension. This pharmacological property persists well into the postoperative period—indeed chlorpromazine has been used to control the postoperative reactionary hypertension that commonly follows major vascular surgery.

Perhaps of even more significance is that postoperative recovery in patients who have been deliberately made hypothermic is considerably prolonged as compared with normothermic patients. As a direct consequence, postoperative chest complications are considerably more common in these elderly patients who have been made hypothermic than in equivalent but normothermic patients. It is, therefore, not surprising that with the improvement in the management of patients with acute renal tubular necrosis, many vascular surgeons have requested that induced hypothermia is not used on their patients who are to undergo renal vascular surgery.

PULMONARY EMBOLECTOMY

Pulmonary embolism can range from the trivial to the immediately fatal. Factors affecting the severity of the embolism are the size of the embolus, its position in relation to the pulmonary arterial tree and the age of the patient. In an elderly patient massive pulmonary embolism is likely to be fatal within a few minutes, but in a younger patient such an embolus, although eventually likely to be fatal unless treated vigorously, may not cause immediate death, even when as much as 80% of the pulmonary circulation is obstructed. In such circumstances death, when it does occur, is due to very progressive and severe right ventricular failure, which can develop at any time within the first 24 hours of the embolism. If the patient is developing right-sided heart failure, then this time is too short for the various medical approaches, such as the use of the different clot-lysing agents even if they are perfused directly into the pulmonary artery.

This has led to a renaissance in the surgical treatment of massive pulmonary embolism. A variety of different surgical approaches is now available. Many involve the use of cardiopulmonary by-pass techniques and as such are outside the scope of this book. There is, though, one technique that does not need cardiopulmonary by-pass methods and technically is not a particularly difficult operation for a competent vascular or thoracic surgeon (Clarke and Abrams, 1972). Its virtues are that once the decision has been made to operate the delays attending organizing and establishing cardiopulmonary by-pass are avoided and the embolus can be removed very quickly. The essentials of the operation are: through a median sternotomy the circulation is deliberately stopped by snaring the vena cava, the pulmonary artery is then opened and the clot lifted out of the artery. Following the removal of the clot, a side clamp is placed over the pulmonary artery incision and the caval snares are released. The circulation automatically restarts. Thereafter the surgeon can close the pulmonary artery at leisure. The total period of complete circulatory occlusion is less than 4 min.

From the anaesthetist's viewpoint these patients are acutely and very severely ill with rapidly distending neck veins of fulminating right ventricular failure. They have a modest degree of cyanosis, mainly stagnant hypoxaemia due to a very low cardiac output and poor peripheral perfusion. Tachycardia and a moderate hypotension with a narrow pulse pressure are usually present. Angiography may show that the patient is surviving by perfusing one branch only of a pulmonary artery, all other branches being totally occluded. The patients are commonly severely agitated and acutely anxious with a marked sense of impending doom.

Physiologically all the reduced cardiac output is flowing through one lobe or worse, through only a few segments of one lobe of one lung. In this zone the blood arriving is very desaturated and is flowing at very high velocity. The zone is very engorged and may be oedematous. The red-cell transit time within the alveolus is substantially reduced, to the point where if the alveolus contains oxygen at a normal partial pressure there may be insufficient time for complete red-cell oxygenation (the oxygenation time is a function of the degree of venous blood desaturation, the alveolar–venous blood oxygen tension gradient and the red-cell transit time as well as the degree of alveolar oedema if this should be present). As a result of the engorgement some degree of intrapulmonary shunting of venous blood also occurs. The arterial oxygen tension, when the patient is breathing air, is low but it will respond to an increase in the inspired oxygen concentration (which increases the size of the alveolar–venous oxygen tension gradient and therefore the alveolar driving diffusive pressure gradient). The engorgement of the pulmonary artery stimulates the respiratory centre so that there is a marked tachypnoea and a significant hypocapnia despite a very substantial increase in deadspace volume, particularly of the parallel deadspace. Another component of the hypoxia is the consequence of the differential changes in regional pulmonary compliance, so that the ischaemic zone of the lung is more compliant than the hyperaemic zone. This, in turn, favours ventilation towards the ischaemic zone. There may also be some Pendeluft ventilation (air swinging from side to side within the chest, like a pendulum, but this air will have a lowered oxygen concentration) because of this variation in regional compliance. The low cardiac output combined with the hypoxaemia induces a moderate metabolic acidosis which progressively increases with time. However, the major physiological event is the reduction in cardiac output. This induces a marked peripheral vasoconstriction which is maintained by considerable over-activity of the vasomotor centre. The situation is then analogous to the young severely injured hypovolaemic patient. Both are exquisitely sensitive to anaesthetic induction agents and readily develop a profound hypotension at the slightest over-dose. However, in the case of pulmonary embolism the cardiac output and blood pressure cannot be restored by further transfusion, as can be achieved in the young injured patient.

There is one other physiological point which has profound implications in the practical aspects of clinical management. These patients have an extremely slow arm–brain circulation time. This time can exceed 3 min. This affects the induction of anaesthesia very considerably, and in two ways. The first is that at induction of anaesthesia there is a very considerable temptation to give too much induction agent as the patient remains awake for so long. The second is the difficulty in applying cricoid pressure at the right time.

The principles of clinical management are therefore straightforward.

Induction

Anaesthesia should be induced with the patient already on the operating table and the surgeon scrubbed up ready. An intravenous infusion line is established and the ECG electrodes are attached. An assistant or nurse is assigned to monitor the pulse continuously. The dose of all drugs that act on the brain should be drastically reduced until a normal cardiac output has been restored. In practice, this means halving the normal dose of induction agent. Full time allowance should be made for the slow circulation time. Whilst waiting for the induction agent to exert its slow effect the patient should be given oxygen-enriched air, if not 100% oxygen, to breathe and this should be continued until the patient is ready to be intubated. No attempt should be made to ventilate the patient prior to intubation. These are emergency patients and should be presumed to have something in their stomachs. Because of the slowness of the circulation and the lightness of the anaesthesia, no attempt should be made to exert cricoid pressure; its arousal properties are too strong. The induction agent should be given slowly. During the administration of the induction agent a large dose of short-acting muscle relaxant should be given, whilst the patient is still fully conscious, and this is followed by the rest of the induction agent. This means that the dose of induction agent must be predetermined, but it ensures the quickest onset of relaxation.

If, as a result of the induction agent, the pulse disappears or the ECG shows a cardiac arrest, the surgeon is asked to open the chest urgently and remove the obstruction in the pulmonary outflow and then to perform open cardiac massage. (External cardiac massage is useless in the situation of a cardiac arrest in massive pulmonary embolism.) Meanwhile the trachea is rapidly intubated and the patient ventilated with 100% oxygen. If the pulse pressure remains, the patient is rapidly intubated and ventilated and a radial artery is cannulated. Not too much time should be spent on arterial cannulation, although an arterial line will be useful for subsequent monitoring of the degree of metabolic acidosis which develops during the period of total circulatory standstill.

Thereafter the operation proceeds apace. Once the caval snares are applied, the anaesthetist should keep track of the passing time and alert the surgeon when 3 min have elapsed. After the circulation has been restored, intravenous analgesics can be given, preferably morphine or one of its derivatives, as these produce the minimum disturbance of haemodynamics. Five or more minutes after restoration of the circulation some assessment should be made of the degree of acid–base disturbance, although 50 mmol of sodium bicarbonate can be given empirically. If the patient's condition allows, then following induction and arterial cannulation, a central venous catheter should be inserted. This is not usually a difficulty as the patient already has distended neck veins, but again not too much time should be spent on this, and an external jugular cannulation will be every bit as informative as an internal jugular cannulation. Following release of the pulmonary obstruction, the central venous pressure should slowly fall. If the right ventricle has been grossly over-distended, or the central venous pressure remains persistently high coupled with a persistently low arterial pressure, the patient may need some inotropic support to maintain the cardiac output.

Thereafter the patient is managed like any other thoracotomy patient, complete with chest drains.

Postoperative care

The principal problem in postoperative management lies in the quality of function of the right ventricle. If the right ventricle recovers quickly from the stress to which it has been subjected, then postoperative management is very simple and follows that of any thoracotomy. If the right ventricle is sluggish, then inotropic agents will need to be sustained for some time and all motor activity reduced to a minimum, including respiration. The patient should be ventilated with a flow-cycled, pressure-limited ventilator as this type of ventilator produces the minimum disturbance of intrapulmonary haemodynamics (Cournand et al., 1948).

There are three other prime components of postoperative care following a successful pulmonary embolectomy: (1) Pain, which needs intravenous narcotics, of which by far the best choice is morphine because of its beneficial effects on pulmonary artery pressure (Vismara et al., 1976). (2) Acid–base balance, which means frequent arterial blood gas analyses and titrating alkali until normal blood gas values are obtained. (3) Urinary output, which is likely to need diuretics. If the central venous pressure is very high, the patient may need a forced diuresis to lower the central venous pressure and thereby make the right ventricular function more efficient.

Pulmonary embolism rarely arises *de novo*. Usually there is a precipitating cause such as deep vein thrombosis following trauma, which may be surgical. In the general bustle of treating the pulmonary embolus the treatment of the underlying cause should not be forgotten. This applies particularly to trauma victims who may have damaged joints which need sustained and vigorous treatment to prevent permanent disability from intracapsular adhesions and joint fibrosis. The question of subsequent anticoagulants and/or antibiotics should be discussed with the surgical team.

Brain damage

During the period of partial pulmonary occlusion and reduced cardiac output the brain, as one of the essential organs, will have received a blood flow that will maintain normal brain function. Indeed, the patient is often fully conscious and only too aware of what is happening. Providing that the arterial blood up to the time of total circulatory occlusion is fully oxygenated, the patient can withstand 4 or so minutes of elective cardiac standstill whilst anaesthetized without developing brain damage. If the patient is hypoxaemic or severely hypotensive prior to the elective cardiac standstill, this time is eroded. Nevertheless, patients have survived without permanent brain damage periods of time of total circulatory occlusion against a background of hypoxaemia and hypotension which were considerably in excess of 4 min (Tomlin et al., 1981). However, there is likely to be a period of considerable cerebral oedema with the patient partially comatose, perhaps passing through a period of spasticity, hemiplegia and cortical blindness before making a full recovery. It may take as long as a week for the patient to pass through these stages and total recovery of all brain function may not be achieved for several months. Thus if after the pulmonary embolectomy the patient appears severely brain damaged the outlook is not totally gloomy, and any prognosis given should be extremely guarded.

DISSECTING ANEURYSMS

In contrast to the situation of massive pulmonary embolism, where very aggressive surgery can be very beneficial, the results of surgery for dissecting aneurysms have been very disappointing. Without aggressive treatment 84% of patients, with dissecting aneurysms of all types, die within 6 weeks, most are dead within the first few days (Hirst et al., 1958). Dissecting aneurysms are graded into one of three types. The first two types involve either aneurysms arising in the ascending aorta with perhaps some pericardial involvement or even tamponade, or those that arise in the arch of the aorta. If surgery is contemplated these two types require the full facilities of cardiopulmonary by-pass and as such are beyond the scope of this book. In these two types of dissection the patient's only hope is surgery. Attempting to treat these patients by aggressive medical means results in a mortality of 83% (Dalen et al., 1980).

The third type is dissecting aneurysm of the descending aorta. The tear in the intima usually occurs immediately distal to the origin of the left subclavian artery. This type of dissecting aneurysm is rare relative to the other types of dissecting aneurysm, although Dalen and his co-workers (1980) found that 40% of their cases of dissecting aneurysm were of this type. Without aggressive treatment 50% of these patients will die (Lindsay and Hurst, 1975). Wheat and colleagues (1973) noted that the surgical results, with a 25% mortality, were poor and pioneered the aggressive use of hypotensive agents as an alternative to surgery. They claimed that the mortality fell to 14%. Daily and co-workers (1970) found that their mortality with drug treatment was 20%, whilst Austin and his co-workers (1967) also found that the results of medical treatment for this type of dissecting aneurysm were not that much better than the results from surgery. More recently Dalen and colleagues (1980) found that the mortality with vigorous medical treatment was 43%, whereas the mortality after surgery was 36%. This type of dissection is comparatively rare and the various series are not that large and, therefore, this scatter is not significant. Clearly though, operative treatment confers no particular benefit so that the idea of surgical correction is being steadily abandoned in favour of very vigorous hypotensive therapy.

The surgical approach is similar to that of other supradiaphragmatic aneurysms. Either the area of the dissection is resected and replaced with a large Dacron graft or else the aorta at the zone of dissection is firmly enclosed in a stiff plastic sheath to prevent the adventitia from distending further, and in the hope that the blood within the aneurysm will clot and fibrose. Occasionally, the surgeon will attempt a refenestration into the lumen of the aorta at the lowest level of the aneurysm thereby imitating nature's rare method of cure. The result is a double aorta. Providing an escape route for the blood within the aneurysm is no guarantee that all the blood will flow through it, and in the majority of instances the aneurysm continues its dissection and eventual terminal rupture.

During the operation an essential part is the setting up of a temporary by-pass graft between the circulation to the upper half of the body and the lower half. This relieves any mechanical stress on the myocardium when the descending aorta is cross-clamped, and maintains perfusion to the bowel, liver and kidneys. A key aspect of the anaesthetic management is to avoid any burst of hypertension until such time as the aorta is cross-clamped, otherwise the aneurysm may dissect further and rupture. This applies to the act of intubation as well as to the time of skin incision. Since these patients often have associated ischaemic heart disease, an anaesthetic technique of deliberate hypotension is not without its dangers.

The anaesthetic principles involved are intubation, muscle relaxation and controlled ventilation, analgesia by intravenous narcotics and blood pressure controlled by the judicious use of rapidly acting inhalational agents. The operation involves a thoracotomy, but a double-lumen tube is unnecessary, and possibly is contra-indicated because of the disturbance in blood pressure that may accompany its insertion. It must be presumed that the whole surface of the lumen of the aorta is friable and likely to tear, so that even after the aneurysm has been dealt with, hypertension must be avoided in case another dissection results. This applies particularly to extubation, with the coughing or straining that may ensue, as well as to the immediate postoperative period.

Even if the patient survives the surgery, the postoperative problems are immense. These are: postoperative chest infection, atelectasis and lung collapse, haemothorax, pneumothorax, myocardial infarction, oesophageal malfunction, including complete oesophageal ulceration and necrosis due to obstruction and occlusion of the feeding arteries to the oesophagus, mediastinitis, redissection of the aneurysm, haemorrhage from the anastomotic site, renal failure due either to acute tubular necrosis or to renal artery thrombosis—the latter being in turn due to either the dissection extending to encircle the origin of the renal arteries and compressing them until they thrombose or to primary thrombosis as a result of hypotension. But the greatest danger is paraplegia from spinal artery occlusion. These patients are very poor clinical material and it is small wonder that the results are so bad.

The medical management should take place in an intensive care unit. The patients will need to be on controlled hypotension for several days. This control must be very exact and requires arterial cannulation and continuous monitoring on an oscilloscope, preferably recorded as a trend on a very slow pen recorder. Alpha-blocking agents are then given and the response noted. Unfortunately, the initial response is variable and even if good control of blood pressure is obtained tachyphylaxis frequently develops within 24–48 hours. Continuous infusions of sodium nitroprusside have been tried, but these cannot be sustained for too long because of toxicity problems related to the accumulation of the metabolic breakdown products of sodium nitroprusside, such as thiocyanate and cyanide (Pharmaceutical Codex, 1979b). Infusions of trinitrate have also been used but again adaptation or tachyphylaxis may occur. Small doses of beta-blocking drugs can also be used, but occasionally against the background of peripheral vasodilators the hypotension can be very severe.

Meanwhile, the patient goes into a state of autonomic confusion with gut stasis, possible ileus and fluid loss, and bladder dysfunction. Nutrition then becomes a problem. The patient must be nursed in bed with a head-up tilt, and if he sags into the horizontal position the blood pressure rises as the venous pooling effect is negated. An attempt is made to maintain the controlled hypotension for at least a week in the hope that the dissection will not extend and the blood in the aneurysmal sac will clot and fibrose. Meanwhile it is hoped that the intimal tear heals. Occasionally, but only occasionally, it does.

REFERENCES

Atkinson R. S., Rushman G. B. and Lee J. A. (1982a) Hypothermia. In: *Synopsis of Anaesthesia*, 9th edn., p. 345. Wright PSG, Bristol

Atkinson R. S., Rushman G. B. and Lee J. A. (1982b) Hypothermia. In: *Synopsis of Anaesthesia*, 9th edn., p. 348. Wright PSG, Bristol

Atkinson R. S., Rushman G. B. and Lee J. A. (1982c) Hypothermia. In: *Synopsis of Anaesthesia*, 9th edn., p. 349. Wright PSG, Bristol

Austin W. G., Buckley M. J. and McFarland J. (1967) Therapy of dissecting aneurysms. *Arch. Surg.* **95**, 835

Clarke D. B. and Abrams L. D. (1972) Pulmonary embolectomy with venous inflow occlusion. *Lancet* **i**, 767

Cournand A., Motley H. L., Werko L. et al. (1948) Physiological studies of the effects of intermittent positive pressure breathing on cardiac output in man. *Am. J. Physiol.* **152**, 162

Crawford E. S. and Rubio P. A. (1973) Reappraisal of adjuncts to avoid ischemia in the treatment of aneurysms of descending aorta. *J. Thorac. Cardiovasc. Surg.* **66**, 693

Crawford E. S., Snyder D. M., Cho G. M. et al. (1978) Progress in treatment of thoraco-abdominal aortic aneurysms involving coeliac, superior mesenteric and renal arteries. *Ann. Surg.* **188**, 404

Daily P. O., Trueblood H. W., Stinson E. B. et al. (1970) Management of acute aortic dissections. *Ann. Thorac. Surg.* **10**, 237

Dalen J. E., Pape L. A., Chan L. H. et al. (1980) Dissection of the aorta: pathogenesis, diagnosis and treatment. *Prog. Cardiovasc. Dis.* **23**, 237

Dunbar R. W. (1979) Thoracic aneurysms. In: *Cardiac Anaesthesia*, vol. 1. p. 369. Editor: Kaplan J. A. Grune & Stratton, New York

Friedman S. M., Johnson R. L. and Friedman C. L. (1954) The pattern of recovery of renal function following renal artery occlusion in the dog. *Circ. Res.* **2**, 231

Gore I. and Hirst A. E. (1973) Arteriosclerotic aneurysms of the abdominal aorta, a review. *Prog. Cardiovasc. Dis.* **16**, 113

Hirst A. E. and Gore I. (1973) Marfan's syndrome: A review. *Prog. Cardiovasc. Dis.* **16**, 187

Hirst A. E., Johns V. J. and Kime S. W. (1958) Dissecting aneurysm of the aorta: a review of 505 cases. *Medicine* **37**, 217

Lindsay J. and Hurst J. W. (1975) Clinical features and prognosis in dissecting aneurysms of the aorta: a reappraisal. *Circulation* **35**, 880

Maclean D. and Emslie-Smith D. (eds.) (1977) The abnormal physiology of hypothermia: metabolic rate. In: *Accidental Hypothermia*, p. 77. Blackwell Scientific Publications, Oxford

Pharmaceutical Codex (1979a) *Chlorpromazine*, p. 184. Pharmaceutical Society of Great Britain. Pharmaceutical Press, London

Pharmaceutical Codex (1979b) *Sodium Nitroprusside*, p. 833. Pharmaceutical Society of Great Britain. Pharmaceutical Press, London

Rob C. and De Weese J. A. (eds.) (1979) Treatment of arterial aneurysms. In: *Operative Surgery: Fundamental International Techniques*. 3rd edn., p. 78. Butterworth, London

Roberts W. C. (1979) Congenital cardiovascular disorders silent until adulthood. In: *Congenital Heart Disease in Adults*, p. 443. Davis, Philadelphia

Samaan H. A. (1971) Hazards of radial artery pressure monitoring. *J. Cardiovasc. Surg.* **12**, 342

Stoney R. J. and Wylie E. J. (1973) Surgical management of arterial lesions of the thoraco-abdominal aorta. *Am. J. Surg.* **126**, 157

Tomlin P. J., Martin C. W. and Honisberger L. (1981) Brain Death: Retrospective surveys. *Lancet* **i**, 378

Tomlin P. J., Schlobaum R., Carson S. A. A. et al. (1966) The effects of hypercapnia, pH and hypothermia on cardiac output in the halothane anaesthetized dog. *Br. J. Anaesth.* **41**, 660

Turney S. Z., Attar S., Ayella R. et al. (1976) Traumatic rupture of the aorta. *J. Thorac. Cardiovasc. Surg.* **72**, 727

Vismara L. A., Leaman D. M. and Zelis R. (1976) The effects of morphine on venous tone in patients with acute pulmonary edema. *Circulation* **54**, 335

Walter J. B. and Israel M. S. (1979) Thrombosis in arteries: atherosclerosis. In: *General Pathology*, 5th edn., p. 496. Churchill Livingstone, London

Wheat R. W., Harris P. D., Malin R. J. et al. (1973) Treatment of dissecting aneurysms. *Prog. Cardiovasc. Dis.* **16**, 87

CHAPTER 8

After-care Following Abdominal Vascular Surgery

Studies on deaths following all forms of anaesthesia and surgery have shown that a significant cause of mortality, occurring in the first week from the start of an anaesthetic, is heart disease, and that ischaemic heart disease accounted for no less than one-third of all deaths (Lunn and Mushin, 1982). It is perhaps significant that, among vascular surgery patients, ischaemic heart disease is much more prevalent than it is in the normal population. Just on half of the deaths (52·3%), in that first week, occurred in ordinary wards and one-third of the deaths occurred in the first 24 hours.

Against this background vascular surgery is high-risk surgery. Twenty years ago the mortality after elective surgery for infrarenal aortic abdominal aneurysms was 10%, ten years ago it was about 5%. This improvement is largely due to improved postoperative care. Nowadays an uncomplicated elective aneurysm resection carries with it a mortality rate of around 3% (Tomlin, 1978). This is as high as that after elective open heart surgery. This rate doubles with every additional disease present or that develops, and vascular patients frequently have other diseases present. Emergency aortic surgery has a mortality rate that ranges from 37% to 69%, with a mean of 54% (Gore and Hirst, 1973). The overwhelming bulk of this mortality occurs postoperatively. The mortality rate is very high in the initial postoperative period but then falls off exponentially, but about 80% of all the postoperative deaths among vascular surgery patients occur in the first 10 postoperative days.

Patients who have undergone major vascular surgery involving extensive abdominal dissection should be cared for in an intensive care unit for at least the first 24 hours after their operation. An important cause of mortality is inadequate postoperative supervision by hard-pressed but relatively inexperienced nursing staff trying to cope with not only the vascular patient but all the other patients in a busy surgical ward. It is quite absurd that very highly trained staff should spend many hours performing very skilled and complex work in surgery, in resuscitation and in patient care only for it all to be of no avail because of inadequate after-care on the ward. This problem is at its most acute at night. This does bring into question whether establishments which do not have appropriate after-care facilities should undertake this kind of work, even as an emergency.

As far as the intensive care unit is concerned, there may also be a genuine conflict of pressure on the staff when looking after a vascular patient since much of the attention they provide appears minor and relatively trivial as compared with, say, looking after a patient who has undergone cardiopulmonary by-pass surgery. This can lead to serious questioning of the need for postoperative intensive care for vascular patients. Yet the prophylactic value of such attention, though superficially it may appear trivial, cannot be underestimated. When this prophylactic care is given, there are very considerable improvements, not only in mortality and survival but also in morbidity (Tomlin, 1978).

The immediate after-care for patients who have undergone major vascular surgery conveniently splits into two major divisions. These are: (a) those concerned with local problems arising from the surgery itself—haemorrhage, graft clotting, embolization etc.—all of which are likely to need further surgery, and (b) the general problems arising out of total patient care. These general problems can then be classified under a number of separate headings. No one heading is all-important and a disorder of any one of them potentially is a potent source of major morbidity, if not mortality, in these high-risk patients.

The principal areas of concern are:

Analgesia
Respiratory care
Controlled ventilation
Circulatory after-care
Electrolyte imbalance
Hepatic and renal problems
Metabolic and nutritional support
Energy considerations

ANALGESIA

The surgical incision for an intra-abdominal vascular operation is a long one. The skin incision frequently extends from the xiphisternum to just above the symphysis pubis. In addition, there is usually very extensive dissection of the peritoneum of the posterior abdominal wall. All these areas are highly sensitive and are sources of much postoperative pain. The analgesic requirements initially will depend upon what has been used by the anaesthetist during the operation. But whatever has been used, eventually there will be a need for additional analgesics in the postoperative period. The duration of severe postoperative pain, of sufficient intensity as to require powerful narcotics to subdue it, is 4–6 days. With other vascular operations that do not involve the abdomen or thorax, e.g. femoral–popliteal by-pass surgery or carotid artery surgery, the duration of severe postoperative pain is very much less, commonly only one or two days.

There are two principal reasons why good analgesia is necessary. The first is the humane one, to relieve suffering. Whilst any analgesia is better than none, yet there is a strong tendency to minimize this aspect of patient care, usually because of a misplaced anxiety that too much narcotic, for this period of time, might turn the patient into a narcotic addict. A number of these patients are elderly, somewhat stoical and reluctant to worry busy nursing staff until the pain becomes unbearable. So they suffer in silence. The second principal reason is to counter the adverse physiological consequences of pain.

As far as oxygen homeostasis and breathing are concerned, there are three specific physiological consequences of pain:

(1) It induces hypoxaemia in its own right. All patients in pain, irrespective of cause, become hypoxaemic. If the pain arises from areas not involved in respiratory movement, the hypoxaemia will be accompanied by hypocarbia. Thus the hypoxaemia is due to a ventilatory perfusion ratio imbalance rather than defective ventilation. The interrelation between pain, age and Pao_2 is that the regression line relating age and Pao_2 in patients in pain, but who have not been operated upon, is below but parallel to that of preoperative patients who are free from pain (Phillips and Tomlin, 1977). That is to say, pain makes its own specific contribution to hypoxaemia that summates with the age response (Nunn, 1965; Bay et al., 1968; Marshall and Wyche, 1972; Nunn, 1981a). The ventilation–perfusion ratio imbalance persists even during any postoperative artificial ventilation. The mechanism by which pain produces this effect is obscure.

(2) Pain induces reflex muscle rigidity as part of a general response to reduce movement of the painful areas. As far as the patients who have undergone abdominal vascular surgery are concerned, this means tightening of the abdominal wall, thereby opposing descent of the diaphragm. There is, therefore, more intercostal movement, which is physically tiring in the subject unused to intercostal breathing. As the intercostal muscles fatigue so ventilation becomes reduced. It may take up to 15 hours before the intercostal muscles fatigue to the point whereby the patient starts developing carbon dioxide retention.

(3) Despite the use of the intercostal muscles the respiratory movements induce pain. Automatically the patient attempts to inhibit this movement so that the tidal excursion is reduced and this is

compensated for by a higher frequency of breathing. This rapid shallow breathing is wasteful of effort as the deadspace : tidal volume (VD/VT) ratio deteriorates, and this is a further source of muscle fatigue. Eventually there will be some carbon dioxide retention and respiratory acidosis. A complicating factor is that many of these patients have a mild degree of chronic bronchitis. If there is much pain, sputum retention will develop as it hurts to cough. This, in turn, will lead to marked pulmonary atelectasis and segmental obstruction, further ventilation–perfusion ratio inequalities and a worsening of the hypoxaemia. The atelectases, and there may be more than one, will, in turn, induce a mild fever which increases the metabolic rate and oxygen consumption which will worsen any existing hypoxaemia yet further. All these problems take time to develop, up to 18–24 hours.

These adverse physiological consequences account for the curious pattern of morbidity sometimes seen in these patients. This is the phenomenon best described as a 'bright interval'. It is analogous to the 'silent interval' after the onset of peritonitis following a perforation of a peptic ulcer, or the 'lucid interval' after a head injury; that is, after a period of moderate well-being the patient deteriorates rapidly. In the vascular patient this pattern is that in the first few hours after surgery the patient appears well—very well; so well that he may be prematurely discharged from the intensive care unit to the ordinary ward. Postoperative analgesia is then perhaps not as good as it should be. The adverse respiratory consequences develop, and gradually lead up to a severe postoperative chest problem with respiratory failure. This progressive deterioration eventually necessitates urgent readmission to the intensive care unit on the third to fourth postoperative day. Herein lies the difference between the general surgical patient who has had a laparotomy or gastrectomy. By the third or fourth postoperative day his pain is diminishing substantially. Such patients are then better able to cope with any respiratory difficulties and are able to cough more effectively. As a result, postoperative frank respiratory failure, although it does occur in general surgical patients, is much less common. It is the persistence of severe postoperative pain in vascular surgery patients that is the nub of the problem.

There has been much recent effort to combat the problem of postoperative pain. These efforts have ranged from frequent intravenous administrations of narcotic to constant infusions of narcotics by means of dedicated syringe pumps (Chakravarty et al., 1979). Postoperative pain is not a static thing but varies in intensity with time, waxing and waning every few hours, with considerable variation in this fluctuation between patients (Gjessing and Tomlin, 1979). This, in turn, provides the physiological basis of a variety of self-administration systems (Welchew, 1983) by which the patient, subject to certain safeguards, is able to control the rate of infusion of narcotic from the syringe pump or infusion system (White et al., 1979). This approach is not entirely apposite to the elderly vascular patient who may be confused (which could be one result of the hypoxaemia) or have mild senility. Elderly patients are also unduly susceptible to the respiratory depressant effects of narcotics. Dosage is normally calculated on a weight basis, but this can lead to an overdose in the obese elderly patient. The laryngeal protective reflexes are depressed following surgery, and may be further depressed by narcotics. Narcotics are also powerful emetics, so that there is a small but definite risk of the patient developing an acid aspiration syndrome.

An alternative approach to the question of pain control is to use local anaesthetics. Since the pain is long-lasting, the only practical technique of using local anaesthetics is by continuous epidural analgesia. This is not really applicable to vascular surgery patients because of the disturbance of the autonomic control of blood pressure which epidurally applied local anaesthetics produce. Apart from the question of the effects that a continuous epidural local anaesthetic can have on the haemodynamics in an elderly arteriopathic patient, the quality of supervision, top ups, etc. and the duration for which this regimen must be sustained render the use of epidurally applied local anaesthetic drugs as inappropriate. There is no substitute for narcotics.

This leads to the question of epidural narcotics. Epidural narcotics have a biphasic system of absorption from the epidural space. The first phase is systemic vascular absorption of narcotic from the epidural space. The extent of this is uncontrollable. If the epidural space is hyperaemic, all the narcotic will be absorbed systemically; the effect is then the same as an intramuscular injection of narcotic (Chambers et al., 1981). However, the dose of narcotic given epidurally is usually less than the dose of an intramuscular injection, and so the patient will have inadequate analgesia. An example of this is the use of epidural morphine in the woman in labour (Husemeyer et al., 1980). The second phase is dural absorption, whereby the narcotic is absorbed through the dura into the cerebrospinal fluid. This is a much slower process than systemic absorption and the amount of narcotic absorbed will depend mainly on how much of the drug is left after the systemic absorption phase. There is a reduced vascularity of the epidural space in the elderly and so there will be proportionately more narcotic absorbed through the dura in the elderly than in the middle aged. Furthermore, the elderly are much more susceptible to the quantity of morphine within the cerebrospinal fluid (Gjessing and Tomlin, 1981). In particular, the elderly, in response to morphine, are more likely to have periods of apnoea than are the younger patients (Arunasalam et al., 1983). Since the intrathecal dose of narcotic is also less than the epidural dose, among the elderly patients there is a real risk that excessive dural absorption of narcotic—combined with the sensitivity to narcotics that elderly patients have—will produce the effects of an over-dose. There is one other problem related to the use of epidural narcotics. Occasionally there is little to no systemic absorption (and so no reasonably rapid metabolism) of the drug. Then all the epidural narcotic rather rapidly passes through into the cerebrospinal fluid. Since the customary dose of epidural narcotic is one and a half to two times the dose of intrathecal narcotic, this excess transference into the cerebrospinal fluid can lead to a very severely narcotized patient. The incidence of this problem would appear to be between 0·5% and 2% of all patients given epidural narcotics.

Intrathecal narcotics, although capable of producing extremely good analgesia, suffer from certain disadvantages (Morgan, 1982). The major one is delayed respiratory depression. It can occur 6 to 12 hours after the intrathecal administration. It is slow in onset, slow to develop and easy to detect providing regular and frequent counts are made of the respiratory rate. This should not be a problem in a well-run intensive care unit.

Another and more distressing problem can occur in the first 2 hours on recovery from the anaesthetic. It is a problem related only to those patients who have had intraperitoneal surgery and who have not had any belladonna derivative, atropine or hyoscine, as a premedicant. Following reversal of the muscle relaxants these patients can develop very intense colic although there is very good parietal analgesia. This problem is discussed in detail in Chapter 4. Intravenous narcotics, particularly pethidine, will block the perception of pain produced by this neostigmine-induced bowel contraction. If the operation lasts for more than 3–4 hours enough of the intrathecal narcotic will have reached the brain to block this perception of pain. Fortunately, most patients become amnesic of the colic episode.

Another disadvantage of intrathecal morphine is more social than medical. Intrathecal morphine provides excellent analgesia for 36–48 hours depending upon the dose. When it does wear off, the patient starts feeling pain, which gradually builds up in intensity over 3–4 hours, with visceral pain occurring before somatic pain. To the patient this pain is remote from the operation, and from being unexpectedly and appreciatively totally analgesic he is now experiencing severe pain. Naturally he will interpret this as a new pain heralding some serious complication. Specific education and reassurance are necessary when this happens. The intrathecal morphine can also be repeated.

Good quality analgesia, however produced, minimizes the stress response to surgery (George et al., 1974; Stanley et al., 1979; Enquist et al., 1980; Christensen et al., 1982; Child and Kaufman, 1985; Hakanson et al., 1985), reduces the excess antidiuretic hormone production (Bonnet et al., 1982; Korinek et al., 1985) and reduces the excess urinary excretion of cortisol, catecholamines and nitrogen (Hjortso et al., 1985) that are features of all major surgery. Postoperatively, this produces a different clinical picture for the attending surgical staff, who may need advising on the changed pattern of postoperative requirements for fluids and electrolytes (Gordon et al., 1973; Kehlet et al., 1979; Twigley and Hillman, 1985).

For some vascular surgery patients the benefits of the newer forms of analgesia may not be appropriate e.g. patients with diabetic neuropathy where it is unwise to perform spinal injections, or emergency cases such as ruptured aortic aneurysms. These patients must, perforce, be treated along more traditional lines, either by periodic injections of analgesic or by the use of constant infusion pump systems. It is a mistake when treating these patients to be too sparing with the analgesics whilst the patient is in the intensive care unit, given the quality of nursing supervision that one should expect, and the easy availability of specific antidotes if any patient should prove to be unduly sensitive to the narcotic.

RESPIRATORY CARE

As a result of abdominal vascular surgery the patient usually has an extensive surgical wound. If this wound is painful, the normal reflex responses to pain inhibit full relaxation of the abdominal muscles so that effortless breathing becomes more difficult. If there is very much pain, this effect is not only compounded by the muscle splinting to pain, described in the previous section, but also by the hypoxaemia produced by pain. Two other factors may be present to inhibit normal blood gas homeostasis. These are: (a) the degree of circulatory instability that has occurred either during surgery or postoperatively, and (b) the background medical status of the patient such as age and its effects on hypoxaemia (Marshall and Wyche, 1972), the presence of other diseases such as chronic bronchitis and emphysema, obesity, hypertension or subclinical left ventricular failure.

Following vascular surgery the patients are hypoxaemic. The extent of this is varied but a Pao_2 much above 11 kPa (80 mmHg) when breathing air is very unusual. Even when there is total analgesia the Pao_2 is lower than that predicted by the age of the patient. Many studies have shown that following any kind of surgery (Nunn J. F., 1981a) the Pao_2 is lower than that predicted by the age of the patient. The severity of this postoperative hypoxaemia is reduced by more than half if there is total analgesia to the point where the patient can move all muscles freely. The response to additional oxygen supplementation shows that the hypoxaemia is not simply due to maldistribution of the respired gases within the lung, but that there must be also a disturbance of the distribution of blood flow within the pulmonary circulation, leading to ventilation–perfusion ratio inequalities, as well as an increase in the absolute shunted fraction of the venous blood in the lungs. Increasing the inspired oxygen concentration to 50% produces an alveolar arterial oxygen tension gradient of up to 20 kPa (160 mmHg). When the inspired oxygen concentration is varied in steps, the size of the apparent shunt, as calculated using the classic shunt equations, also varies. Nomograms of how much additional oxygen to give in order to produce a normal PaO_2 have proved to be a disappointing guide when looking after these patients. There are too many non-quantifiable other variables. It follows that to be sure that the patient is receiving enough oxygen there is no substitute for periodically measuring the oxygen tension of the arterial blood and titrating the additional oxygen against the results.

Hypercapnia is due to inadequate ventilation which, in turn, is likely to be due to (a) too much postoperative analgesics, (b) pain, (c) a disorder of lung mechanics, particularly if there is any disturbance of the normal co-ordinated function of the respiratory muscles because then chest wall compliance decreases, or (d) background obstructive airways disease which may be acute or chronic.

There is one further and more insidious aspect of postoperative respiratory failure in the patient who has had major abdominal vascular surgery. This is the delayed failure following a bright interval. It seems to occur particularly in those patients who have had emergency vascular surgery, e.g. a threatened or even ruptured aortic aneurysm, but can also occur after elective aortic or aorto-iliac surgery. Following an uneventful operation and anaesthetic and apparently, at least initially, reasonably good analgesia, the blood gas data may be fully acceptable with the patient breathing either air or oxygen-enriched air, so that the patient is discharged from the intensive care unit back to the ward. Yet within 36–48 hours there develops clear manifest respiratory failure necessitating returning the patient to the intensive care unit perhaps for intubation and artificial respiration. Radiologically there may be seen, for the first time in that patient, extensive plate atelectases in both lung fields, but particularly on the right side, suggesting that this is due to an aspiration pneumonitis consequent upon laryngeal incompetence (Tomlin et al., 1965). In addition, there is often a marked hilar flare visible on the chest radiographs. On auscultation coarse râles may be heard scattered widely throughout the lungs. The blood gases show marked hypoxaemia, sometimes with hypercarbia. The source of the problem is a mixture of pain, aspiration pneumonitis and inadequate

postoperative pulmonary physiotherapy, leading to sputum retention, atelectasis, hypoxaemia and the left ventricle starting to fail
secondary to the hypoxaemia.

Although artificial respiration plays a dramatic role in the after-care
of patients who have undergone abdominal vascular surgery, the
proportion of patients who need this is steadily diminishing so that
now only about 20% of patients require such treatment. Two factors
have contributed towards this: improved methods of pain control
and, more significantly, the falling incidence of background chronic
bronchitis and emphysema as a result of the 'clean air' movement and
reduction of environmental pollution. Nevertheless postoperative
respiratory after-care does not end there. These patients still require
intensive pulmonary physiotherapy every 2–4 hours during the day in
order that the bases of the lungs are fully expanded and to get rid of
any retained secretions. They are still hypoxaemic and will need
supplementary oxygen for at least 12 hours, depending upon the
blood gas results. If the sputum is discoloured, antibiotics should be
given at once rather than wait for the bacteriological laboratory
results. The most likely organisms will be of the coliform group and
most probably are due to self-contamination such as inhaling infected
particles from the nasopharynx or oropharynx. However, the surgeon
will also have an interest in the choice of antibiotics as he will be
concerned with intra-abdominal infection. Ischaemia of the bowel
renders transluminal spread of bacteria through the gut wall more
likely. Bacteria, previously harmlessly contained within the gut,
escape and become pathogenic. Hence collaboration with the surgeon
on the choice of antibiotic is essential.

CONTROLLED VENTILATION

The indications for artificial ventilation following vascular surgery
are constantly changing. Certain empirical indications have emerged.
They are simple guide-lines but are also dependent upon the degree
of local support available in other aspects of respiratory after-care.
Thus, if the patient has mild chronic bronchitis but there is a good
pulmonary physiotherapy service, it may not be necessary to institute
artificial ventilation as the physiotherapist will be able to cope. If the
physiotherapy service is poor, it may be safer to institute artificial
ventilation rather than let the patient steadily accumulate his own
secretions.

The empirical indications (the order is without significance) which
the author has found are:

1. Background respiratory insufficiency
2. Failure to regain full consciousness

3. Severe obesity
4. Failure of any other major physiological system
5. Extensive retroperitoneal haematoma formation
6. Intra-operative circulatory instability
7. Massive intra-operative blood transfusion
8. Uncompensated persistent hypercapnia

1. Background respiratory insufficiency

This is a major indication for postoperative artificial ventilation in the vascular surgery patient. Inevitably as a result of the surgery, ventilation will be impaired and this will add to the pre-existing lung disease and can lead to overt respiratory failure. In this group of patients it is important not to lower the $Paco_2$ too much as their cerebral capillaries have become acclimatized to a raised $Paco_2$ level. If the $Paco_2$ is lowered too quickly, there will be intense cerebral vasoconstriction which may lead to intense confusion and disorientation. As has been explained earlier, this risk is worse in the arteriosclerotic patient. Empirically the guide-line is the arterial pH, since it is the pH which determines the optimal activity of most of the body enzymes and therefore intracellular function. If the pH is on the alkaline side of 7·40 (hydrogen ion concentration less than 40 nmol/l) the patient is being over-ventilated, irrespective of his $Paco_2$ level. As part of their accommodation to chronic hypercarbia these patients have, renally, retained bicarbonate, but part of this accommodation process is the cerebral capillaries adjusting directly to the altered carbon dioxide tension. The artificial ventilation should be maintained until the patient has more normal respiratory movements. This usually takes several days.

2. Failure to regain full consciousness

Prolonged unconsciousness whether due to drugs, anaesthesia, hypothermia, shock or even an earlier episode of myocardial standstill is another indication for artificial ventilation. It is essential to have the patient's full cooperation during the postoperative physiotherapy. If consciousness is impaired, coughing and deep breathing will also be impaired. The patient is at risk of developing collapse of his lung bases unless artificial ventilation is instituted. The objective of the artificial ventilation is to favour large tidal volumes at low frequency so that expansion of the base of the lungs is facilitated.

3. Severe obesity

This is another indication for artificial ventilation. The proportion of patients with severe obesity is greater among vascular surgery patients than in other groups of patients. This is because obesity facilitates atheromatous deposition. Postoperative pulmonary complications are much higher in the obese patients. This is due to their diminished chest wall compliance so that their respiratory muscles, particularly the intercostal muscles, fatigue more easily. The artificial ventilation is maintained until their chest wall movements are no longer laboured.

4. Failure of any other major physiological system

If there is failure of any major physiological organ or system, such as the heart, the kidneys etc., it is essential to ensure that there is maximal oxygenation of the arterial blood in order to facilitate recovery of that failing organ. In addition, oxygen consumption of the other tissues should be reduced to a minimum. In the fit healthy individual the oxygen consumed by the respiratory muscles accounts for approximately 5% of the basal oxygen consumption (Campbell et al., 1957; Nunn, 1981b). If the work of breathing increases, e.g. due to an increase in lung water consequent upon the failure of a major physiological system, the proportion of inhaled oxygen necessary for respiration increases. Acute failure of any of the major physiological systems induces ventilation–perfusion ratio inequalities. Reducing the body oxygen consumption improves the oxygen content of the venous return. If some of this blood is effectively shunted through the lung, the mean arterial oxygen tension will be that much the higher than if the venous return was low in oxygen. Failure of the circulatory or the renal system is also likely to precipitate serious disturbances of the circulating blood volume and its distribution. Over-loading of the pulmonary circulation is then particularly likely. This will increase the proportion of blood that has been shunted in the lungs, leading to a worsening of the arterial hypoxaemia. Artificial ventilation with supplemental oxygen will reverse these changes.

5. Extensive retroperitoneal haematoma formation

This is particularly applicable to patients who have suffered a frank rupture of the aorta but equally applies to elective surgery patients if during the operation there have been problems in achieving haemostasis, particularly at the sites of graft anastomoses. Patients who have large retroperitoneal haemotomas are particularly hypoxaemic. Why there should be this association between extensive retroperitoneal haematoma formation and subsequent prolonged inadequate gaseous exchange is obscure. The differences are particularly noticeable when reviewing the results of emergency aortic surgery. Prolonged hypoxaemia is considerably more pronounced in those cases where the aorta has ruptured as compared with those cases where the aorta has undergone sudden and severe painful dilatation but not actually ruptured. The hypoxaemia is not easily improved by simple oxygen therapy and artificial ventilation is required, often for a period of days.

6. Intra-operative circulatory instability

This is another indication for postoperative artificial ventilation. In this case the situation is a little clearer. As a result of the intra-operative circulatory instability, the left ventricle may have become over-stretched and moved to its inefficient part of the Starling ventricular function curve. The lungs then become somewhat water-logged. The pulmonary compliance is poor, the work of breathing is excessive and respiration becomes somewhat laboured and shallow. Tachypnoea also develops. The hypoxaemia intensifies, and this worsens the left ventricular failure until the patient is verging on overt pulmonary oedema. The situation is a mild form of acute over-stretching of the left ventricle occasionally seen during cardiopulmonary by-pass surgery. It takes a very long time for a left ventricle to recover if it has been acutely over-filled.

7. Massive intra-operative blood transfusion

Another indication for postoperative artificial ventilation is following a massive blood transfusion during the operation. If, during the operation, the circulating blood volume has been replaced, the patient is unlikely to have normal blood gas values subsequently. Stored blood contains many micro-aggregates (Tomlin, 1976). These micro-aggregates will obstruct the terminal pulmonary arterioles. Each pulmonary arteriole services a number of capillaries, each of which is destined for one or more alveolae. This, in turn, means that a number of alveolae become non-functioning. More importantly, the cells lining the entrance to those alveolae (Weibel, 1973; Williams and Warwick, 1980) lose their nutritional support, they no longer secrete surfactant. Alveolar collapse then ensues and the alveolar dysfunction will persist for many days. If this is widespread throughout the lungs, the chest radiographs will show a 'snowstorm' in the lung fields. The use of fine-screen or other types of filter down to 40 μ undoubtedly have eased this problem (Reul et al., 1973) although Derrington (1985) has challenged this interpretation. The size of the pulmonary arteriole varies between 20 and 40 μ (Elliot and Reid, 1965; Weibel, 1973) so that filtering the blood with a filter pore size of 20 μ will not significantly improve the situation. It is the nest of capillaries with their associated alveolae all being served by the one blocked arteriole which is the heart of the problem. The use of filters is aimed at protecting that arteriole. It is not, however, the complete answer. Some micro-aggregates are unstable and can easily disaggregate whilst passing through the filter, only to re-form lower down the transfusion line. The amount of micro-aggregates that can be given will depend upon a number of factors. These are the size of the transfusion, the age of the blood, or if there has been any disturbance of the blood during haemo-concentration by plasma-reducing techniques in the laboratory. Suffice it to say that the proportion of patients with significant VA/Q problems is much higher in patients who have had a large transfusion than it is for those in whom the need for blood was much less.

8. Uncompensated persistent hypercapnia

Any persistent hypercapnia should be treated with artificial ventilation until the source has been found and treated. In this way the optimum arterial pH will be maintained, and healing thereby facilitated—acidotic tissues heal poorly.

If it is decided to institute artificial ventilation, then the usual principles of care apply. Providing that there are no undue problems relating to compliance, airways resistance or both the choice of ventilator is immaterial. If there is obstructive airways disease, then a ventilator that delivers a predetermined tidal volume with a falling flow wave (De Almeida, 1975), or has an inspiratory hold facility, is to be preferred. This gives a greater residence time of the fresh gas within the lung, so facilitating gaseous exchange. If there is persistent tachypneoic dyspnoea, a machine capable of being patient-triggered, volume limited, with a falling waveform, is then to be preferred. If there are cardiac problems related to the right ventricle, then a gentle ventilator capable of giving a constant flow, and pressure limited, is to be preferred as offering the minimum disturbance to pulmonary haemodynamics (Cournand et al., 1948). The volumes delivered from such a ventilator are likely to change consequent upon changes in the patient's lung compliance, so that frequent checks on the delivered minute volume are essential.

CIRCULATORY AFTER-CARE

There are four aspects of the circulation which are of immediate significance in the postoperative care of the vascular patient. These are:
1. Hypertension
2. Hypotension

3. Myocardial malfunction
4. Leakage or thrombosis of the graft

1. Hypertension

As has been previously discussed, many vascular surgery patients develop a severe transient hypertension in the immediate postoperative period (Roberts et al., 1977; Landymere et al., 1978). It develops within 15 min from the end of anaesthesia and lasts up to 4 hours. It is unrelated to pain. The severity of the hypertension is worse in patients who have not had any centrally acting depressant, such as intra-operative intravenous narcotics, or who have not had any local anaesthetic block such as an epidural block. It is mediated by a catecholamine release, but what the trigger is for this catecholamine release is not known. Anaesthesia as light as simple nitrous oxide anaesthesia will suppress it. It occurs after surgery on any major artery—carotid, coronary, iliac etc. It is not related to adrenal gland manipulation or transient adrenal gland hypoxaemia or hyperaemia. The associated tachycardia is not very great and this suggests that the hypertension is due to noradrenaline rather than adrenaline release. The extent of the hypertension can be very great, 300–350 mmHg is not uncommon, but the duration of the peak of pressure is usually very short and can be measured in milliseconds, so that the peak pressure is too short-lived to be detected by indirect methods of measuring the blood pressure.

In abdominal vascular surgery because of the size and direction of the sutures and the short period of the peak pressure, the force (pressure × area) is not so great as to rupture the sutures at the anastomotic site. This is in contrast to coronary artery by-pass surgery where the hypertension can precipitate a most dramatic cardiac tamponade and graft dehiscence. In carotid artery surgery the risk is a sudden exposure of a previously protected intra-cranial berry aneurysm to a very high pressure and that rupture occurs, causing a subarachnoid or intra-cerebral haemorrhage. The other effect of the hypertension is to increase the work of the heart. This may precipitate arrhythmias and subendocardial ischaemia, although overt angina is very unlikely. ECG monitoring at this stage may show much disturbance of the R–T phase including up to frank elevation of the S–T segment. This usually improves as the hypertension is brought under control.

In vascular surgery patients the hypertension usually responds to chlorpromazine, but if the pulse of pressure is wide or the pressure not brought down quickly, then either sodium nitroprusside or trimetaphan should be used. Chlorpromazine is somewhat slow and unpredictable in this situation, and if a very rapid response is desired, then an infusion of nitroprusside or trimetaphan should be started immediately. Once the hypertension has been broken, it rarely occurs again, so that any recurrence of a raised blood pressure requires re-evaluation of the patient to identify the cause.

2. Hypotension

This is much more sinister in the immediate postoperative phase. It usually means that the patient is bleeding. In contrast to other groups of patients the arteriosclerotic patients usually develop hypotension early if there is internal haemorrhage. This is due to two factors: the ability to vasoconstrict their arterioles to sustain the blood pressure is poor, many of the arterioles are structurally diseased, and the loss of the diastolic pump provided normally by an elastic aorta. As a result, the systolic pressure is much more volume dependent. Therefore, the rate of blood pressure fall is a rough indication of the rate of bleeding. If there is a lot of oozing through a rather porous graft, the rate of blood pressure drop is slow and the blood pressure can easily be restored by transfusion. Frank haemorrhage at the site of vascular anastomoses produces a sharp fall in blood pressure and requires early surgery. External pressure packing over the anastomotic site, if this is possible, is relatively futile. The clinical significance of hypotension is the danger of renal failure or coronary thrombosis.

A mild form of hypotension may occur when postoperative analgesia is particularly effective, as then the normal hormone production in response to stress is lessened (Gordon et al., 1973; Hjortso et al., 1985). Sodium retention is less and renal diuresis is unusually good. If the surgery has involved much handling of the bowel, fluid will be slowly sequestered into the lumen of the bowel. As a result intravascular volume will fall. Treatment is very simple—the patient needs more crystalloid fluids. The guideline for this is the rate of urinary output.

3. Myocardial malfunction

There are two principal aspects of myocardial malfunction in the vascular patient: dysrhythmias and left ventricular failure. These patients are more likely to have a diseased coronary arterial tree so that isolated ventricular ectopic beats are not uncommon and require little treatment other than supportive (i.e. ensuring that the blood pressure is not unduly disturbed, that there is well-oxygenated blood in the arterial system and that there is no hypercapnia). Multiple ectopic beats, particularly multifocal ventricular extra systoles, may require more aggressive therapy such as a lignocaine infusion. The indication for this is if the dysrhythmia is causing hypotension.

Adrenergic beta-blocking drugs are best avoided because of their depressant effect on myocardial contractility. They may create more problems than they solve, such as hypotension or renal failure. The more selective types of beta-blocking drugs hold promise in this field, but as yet clinical experience with the postoperative vascular patient is insufficient to make any informed judgement.

Left ventricular failure requires very energetic treatment if pulmonary oedema or renal failure is to be avoided. A dopamine infusion, if this does not provoke too severe a tachycardia, coupled with a large dose of frusemide will increase the cardiac output and eliminate the excess fluid, so preventing renal failure. Artificial ventilation with an enriched oxygen supply may be required if the arterial oxygen tension does not improve. Digitalis, digoxin or ouabain—not one is particularly helpful unless there is associated atrial fibrillation. The serum potassium level should be checked in case there is any disturbance of potassium balance which is contributing to the left ventricular failure, although potassium imbalance is rarely a significant factor in the aetiology of this problem among patients with arteriopathy.

4. Leakage or thrombosis of the graft

These require urgent re-evaluation by the surgical team and the role of the anaesthetist is secondary to their judgement.

ELECTROLYTE IMBALANCE

Electrolyte imbalance is not normally a severe problem in the patient who has undergone intra-abdominal vascular surgery, at least not in the immediate postoperative period, or unless there is renal impairment. However, during the surgery there inevitably will have been much manhandling of the bowel and this will induce a partial or complete paralysis of the ileum. This causes progressive fluid and electrolyte sequestration in the bowel. Standard postoperative fluid and salt regimens, as after any major abdominal operation, should be enough to deal with this. These may need to be modified if the quality of analgesia is good (Twigley and Hillman, 1985).

Electrolyte imbalance is treated somewhat empirically. The normal sodium requirement per 24 hours is about 120–200 mmol (mEq) per day, but the amount given should be adjusted according to the urinary losses of the previous 24 hours. Serum levels provide useful but qualitative indicators that the extracellular fluid space is hypo- or hypernatraemic. They do not take into account any loss of sodium to within the cells (e.g. sick cell syndrome), nor the losses into the bowel produced by the paralytic ileus. If the kidneys are working well, then a low urinary output of sodium means that the extracellular space is sodium depleted and the body is trying to conserve sodium. As such this is an indication for increasing the sodium input. Equally, if the urinary output of sodium is high this is an indication that the presumed daily requirement of sodium should be lowered. It is important that, in making these judgements, the sample of urinary output should be from the pooled volume of the whole of the previous 24 hours' output, as there may well have been episodes of diuresis induced by diuretics which would produce a copious but dilute urine. If only samples of this diuresis are taken and analysed, this could give a false picture of the 24-hourly sodium excretion.

Potassium daily requirements are approximately 40 mmol (mEq) per 24 hours. Again the dose is adjusted according to the urinary output of potassium over the previous 24 hours. More attention should be paid to the serum level as intravascular haemolysis can increase the serum concentration of potassium. If a large quantity of blood, particularly old blood, has been used during the transfusion, this could be an important source of the excess potassium. There is also a linear relationship between the serum potassium concentration and the carbon dioxide tension. Hypercapnia can increase the loss of potassium from the cell and hypocapnia will lower the serum potassium (Hassan et al., 1979). If nutrition is being maintained by a potassium–insulin–glucose mixture, then any additional potassium must be tempered against this source of potassium. Under these circumstances the potassium levels should be measured very frequently, 2 hourly if necessary. If there is renal failure, potassium infusion should be very tightly controlled against the serum level.

There is, though, one particular but rare complication which will dramatically disturb the electrolyte and water balance. This is ischaemic colitis, first described by Bernatz (1960). If the mesenteric vessels are already partially occluded by atheroma, the various intraoperative manipulations can render the bowel temporarily totally ischaemic. The colon is particularly vulnerable in this respect. A necrotizing ischaemic colitis, which can vary from a frank but patchy necrosis of the colon epithelium down to widespread and severe epithelial damage in which the epithelium of the entire colon may be shed, is a rare but very serious problem leading to extensive fluid losses and melaena. Intensive fluid support and blood transfusion are necessary but the outlook for the patient is very poor, with a coliform septicaemia a very real secondary hazard.

If there is severe renal impairment, then the fluid and electrolyte therapy should be calculated and treated as separate entities. Fluid volume, conveniently given as 5% dextrose, will have to be titrated against the central venous pressure and the arterial pressure as the circulating blood volume adjusts to the various fluid shifts in and out of the bowel. Electrolytes can then be added, each separately, but frequent estimations of the serum sodium and potassium levels are necessary and the treatment regimen adjusted accordingly.

HEPATIC AND RENAL PROBLEMS

Renal problems are common after vascular surgery, but particularly so after aortic or aorto-iliac surgery, and they make a very significant contribution to surgical mortality. Thus the mortality of patients with a ruptured aortic aneurysm who develop renal failure is over 70%, as compared with only 25% where there is no renal failure (Abbott, 1980). Powis (1975) found that two-thirds of all patients showed some degree of increased renal malfunction following aortic surgery, and this was worse in the patients with a frank rupture of an aortic aneurysm. Pollock and Johnson (1973) also observed significant deterioration of renal function after clamping the infrarenal aorta. Many of these patients are old and already have the renal impairment that commonly occurs in older subjects (Kalchthaler, 1978). The anaesthetist has a useful role in helping to prevent renal failure, in that it has been observed empirically that where there is a generous use of intravenous fluids and good attention to renal output during the operation the incidence and severity of postoperative renal failure are markedly less (Thompson et al., 1968).

Renal failure

There are a number of different factors, any of which can combine to produce renal failure in the arteriosclerotic patient. Among these factors are:

1. Any damage done to the kidney as a result of the degenerative hypertension consequent on an inelastic aorta.
2. Atheromatous occlusion of a renal artery precipitating renal hypertension ('Goldblatt kidney', Goldblatt et al., 1934), leading to permanent renal damage.
3. Multiple minor embolization into the renal arteries arising from cross-clamping the aorta close to the origin of the renal arteries. During the period of cross-clamping the resulting turbulence of the arterial blood can sweep off minor thrombi that have formed on the atheromatous surface of the descending aorta. These thrombi can then enter the renal arteries to cause further renal damage.
4. Severe hypotension from any cause occurring during the anaesthetic period. Renal blood flow is already severely reduced

during aortic surgery (Gamulin et al., 1984) and any intra-operative hypotension will only add to this.

5. If there has been pre-existing marked renal impairment and the patient has received a large blood transfusion so that subsequent haemolysis of this blood produces a jaundice, the excess bilirubin can precipitate a hepato-renal syndrome (Epstein, 1982).

6. The age of the patient: this is the most common of all. Some degree of renal failure is common among the elderly, and arterial surgery patients are more likely than most other groups of patients to show, histologically, the atrophic degenerative changes in the renal architecture which accompany ageing (Kalchthaler, 1978).

It is not surprising therefore that in those centres with a busy vascular surgery commitment, renal failure following aortic aneurys-mectomy is a major indication for acute haemodialysis. In this respect it has replaced septic abortion although the numbers are much less.

During the anaesthetic period the anaesthetist needs to maintain strict supervision on renal function, that is, on urinary output, and, if necessary, give 20–40 mg frusemide during the anaesthetic if the urinary output falls below 30 ml per hour. The same considerations apply to the postoperative period. If the urinary output still does not improve, and assuming that the patient is not hypovolaemic, then the dose of frusemide should be increased substantially (250 mg or more), plus, if necessary, a dilute infusion of dopamine. Dopamine in low doses, 2–5 μg per kg per min, will increase glomerular filtration, renal blood flow and sodium excretion (Weiner, 1980), yet this concentration is below that which produces a positive inotropic effect on the heart. Such an aggressive therapeutic approach will prevent anuria if started early enough, but inevitably will not succeed on every occasion.

If the total anuria does develop, it is necessary to determine whether there is any renal blood flow, as there are two potential causes of anuria. These are (a) acute tubular necrosis and (b) renal artery thrombosis. If the problem is one of acute tubular necrosis, then the patient needs haemodialysis and it may be necessary to continue this for up to 6 weeks. If the problem is that there is no renal blood flow, then there will be no recovery from the renal damage and the choice is one of either permanent haemodialysis with a possible subsequent renal transplant or to withdraw all active therapy. Patients with severe arterial disease are normally considered as poor candidates for renal transplantation. The usual, and technically simpler, alternative to haemodialysis is peritoneal dialysis but this is not appropriate in the arterial surgery patient if the surgery has taken place in the abdomen. This is because of the risk of intraperitoneal infection. In peritoneal dialysis low-grade intraperitoneal infection is common and can usually be contained by antibiotic therapy. The presence of a foreign body, such as the dialysis catheter, makes eradication of the infection much more difficult so that often the dialysis catheter has to be removed temporarily. The presence of another foreign body, in this case the graft material, makes eradication of the infection vastly more difficult. If the graft itself becomes infected, almost invariably it means the death of the patient from either an infected erosion of the aorta at the graft anastomosis or the formation of an aortoduodenal fistula. If there are no facilities for haemodialysis, then an alternative to peritoneal dialysis which has been tried is pleural dialysis (combined with artificial respiration). Although, as a dialysing system, pleural dialysis does work, yet the problems of pleural infection are much greater than peritoneal infection (in the non-vascular patient). As a system it has not found much favour and clinical experience is very limited.

There is one other combination in which renal failure occurs, but happily this is rare in the treatment of vascular surgery patients. This is when the renal failure is part of a more global failure of all major physiological systems. Respiratory failure is the first to develop, then follows renal failure. All too soon circulatory failure develops with a progressive refractory hypotension. Next comes hepatic failure characterized by a deterioration of all indices of hepatic function. The central venous pressure rises, the alveolar arterial oxygen tension gradient widens, the heart progressively fails as does cerebral cortical function. The inspired oxygen concentration has to be increased above levels likely to produce oxygen toxicity effects. If improvement does not occur quickly, pulmonary compliance worsens as the changes of oxygen toxicity start to develop. The patient gradually peters out after a struggle that may last for several days. This is the picture of death from multiple systems failure (Tilney et al., 1973; Baue, 1983). It is often characterized by death but with normal electrolytes and blood gases, particularly if vigorous efforts have been made to correct all deviations from normality as they occur. Whilst intraperitoneal infection, perhaps with septicaemia or graft failure, are common precipitating causes for this syndrome of multiple systems failure yet this is not always the case. It may be that the patient is just too old to cope with the extensive surgery which was needed. This syndrome of multiple systems failure is much more common among those patients undergoing emergency aneurysm resection than among those undergoing elective aneurysm surgery, and this implies that it is a consequence of those physiological changes which occurred during the emergency period.

Pure hepatic problems are rare in vascular surgery unless there has been pre-existing hepatic disease. After very major vascular surgery there is always some impairment of hepatic function with rising transaminase levels and a rising serum bilirubin level. Most of the latter is due to haemolysis of either the transfused blood or the absorbing haematoma. With the associated paralytic ileus the biliary excretion system is less able to excrete the bile and so both the conjugated and non-conjugated forms of bilirubin increase. Very commonly if there is marked hepatic impairment, renal failure develops as part of a hepato-renal syndrome. The kidneys in the vascular surgery patient who has an elevated bilirubin appear to be much more vulnerable to mild degrees of hypotension than if the bilirubin is either normal or only very slightly raised. It would appear that hepatic impairment sensitizes the kidneys to early failure and this sensitization increases if there is already a very mild degree of pre-existing renal impairment. Maintaining good renal function, and normotension, is even more critical if there is any suggestion of hepatic dysfunction.

METABOLIC AND NUTRITIONAL SUPPORT

Metabolic care can be considered under three headings:

1. Oxygen availability
2. Electrolyte balance
3. Nutritional support

1. Oxygen availability

Oxygen supply has been discussed and is reasonably easy to achieve, at least on a short term basis. Tissue hypoxia is reflected by metabolic acidosis. It rarely is a problem in the postoperative vascular surgery patient unless there is something seriously amiss with the graft or the patient has a marked reduction in cardiac output. Treatment of metabolic acidosis is simple: the administration of sodium bicarbonate in divided doses titrated against serial blood gas analyses. If the bicarbonate is given too quickly, there is a danger of an abrupt fall in the ionized calcium. This will lead to a sharp fall in myocardial contractility, severe hypotension and a reduced cardiac output, thereby intensifying the metabolic acidosis. Although this condition is self-limiting, the vascular patient is particularly vulnerable to hypotension with a serious risk of myocardial ischaemia or even coronary thrombosis. If the blood pressure does fall during bicarbonate therapy, the patient should be given calcium intravenously. Calcium chloride acts immediately but calcium gluconate requires passage through the liver for the gluconate moiety to be removed and the calcium to be available in an ionized form. Since it is the calcium ion that is required to treat a low cardiac output state, this means that the passage of the gluconate through the liver will be slow. It will take quite a few minutes before the ionized calcium is available to replace that calcium which has been precipitated out of the circulation by the bicarbonate. Meanwhile the hypotension continues. There is, therefore, no pharmacological logic in preferring calcium gluconate to calcium chloride when dealing with this particular set of circumstances.

2. Electrolyte balance

This has been discussed earlier.

3. Nutritional support

This is not usually necessary for the first few days after vascular surgery unless the patient is previously cachectic as from malnutrition due to senile dementia. In those first few days there is marked catabolism but by the fourth or fifth postoperative day the patient is usually able to take some nutrition, as the ileus should have settled down by then. Up to that time a 5% dextrose infusion will have supplied enough carbohydrate to maintain efficient oxidation of body fat so that keto-acidosis is not a problem. If the patient is an insulin-dependent diabetic, he should be maintained on short-acting insulins whose dose levels should be titrated against the blood sugar or urinary sugar concentration.

Parenteral nutrition and protein turnover

If the patient still needs intensive care support by the end of the fifth day to one week, he will need parenteral nutrition. The best indicator for when to start this is the serum albumin level. When this starts to fall, parenteral nutrition should be initiated. The liver is the major organ for protein and amino-acid metabolism. Under conditions of surgical stress the liver increases its protein turnover. Some of the protein consumed is eventually synthesized to replace the globin portion of haemoglobin, of which there is accelerated synthesis after any major operation. Other parts of the protein consumed are eventually converted into suitable protein, by the bone marrow, for platelet synthesis, which also increases after any major operation. In addition, some protein will be consumed in the synthesis of antibodies to combat any infection or antigens introduced by the surgeon, and to make the protein component of sputum. Not all this new protein is manufactured in the liver, but the breakdown of alternative proteins to provide the essential amino-acids and peptides required by the peripheral tissues such as the bone marrow, the lymph nodes, T-cells, mucous glands etc., to synthesize their particular proteins, this breakdown must take place in the liver. Any large wound also consumes a lot of both thrombin and fibrin. The thrombin is involved in clot formation and the fibrin is used as part of the initial scaffolding of the inflammatory response. Further protein is consumed in the formation of granulation tissue. The precursors of all these come directly from the liver. The liver has a certain amount of stored amino-acids which are initially used in this new protein synthesis. In addition, it will metabolize any unwanted protein to provide further amino-acids and peptide chains. The prime source of this is myoglobin, released as a result of the general inactivity consequent upon bed rest, muscle wasting and general catabolic response which follows any surgery. If there is still an increased demand for amino-acids the liver will use any other protein source that it can which does not immediately imperil the body. The serum albumin, as it floats past the liver cell, is another prime target.

Meeting this increased demand with amino-acid infusions has proved to be somewhat disappointing. Whilst occasionally it checks the rate of fall of serum albumin, it rarely stops it completely. There are two reasons for this. In any period of starvation liver protein synthesis is reduced, but as soon as amino-acids or protein are administered the liver increases its rate of synthesis so that the amino-acid infusion has to meet this increased demand. Another, and perhaps more important, reason lies in the amino-acid mixture. It is rarely balanced to meet the metabolic demands for specific amino-acids of any individual patient. Excessive quantities of non-essential (and easy and cheap to manufacture) amino-acids such as glycine are frequently present. Yap and co-workers (1978) and Kelman and his colleagues (1972) have stressed the importance of the amino-acid tryptophan in this respect. Tryptophan will substitute for a number of other amino-acids, both essential and non-essential (Arias et al., 1982). If there is an excess of glycine, it will be simply used as a fuel source, like glucose. The most logical mixture of amino-acids to give to patients are those derived from the hydrolysis of animal protein such as milk. This will at least contain the various amino-acids in the proportion that exists in protein. Concoctions of synthetic amino-acids mixed together do not always have the amino-acids in the correct proportion.

An alternative way of maintaining the serum level of albumin is to give an infusion of albumin. This will maintain the serum level and improve the oncotic performance of the circulation temporarily, but simple quantitative calculations show that as the serum albumin level rises, so the rate of liver consumption of albumin increases, only to decay as the albumin level falls once more. Albumin infusion does buy time as part of the general protein support of the seriously catabolic patient, and it is to be hoped that in that time the patient will start to improve. Another useful protein source is plasma, although albumin has the advantage of being available in a more concentrated form, up to 20%, which is useful if limitations are necessary on the total volume input because of associated renal failure. The globulin fraction of plasma may have some useful components, fibrinogen and certain antibodies etc., but this is somewhat of a gamble as it will depend upon the origin of the plasma.

It is almost impossible to calculate the quantity of protein, or amino-acids which a patient needs. Basic considerations are that a patient requires 50 g/day for normal metabolism. After any surgical stress the protein requirement, or its nitrogen equivalent, increases sharply, but the extent depends upon the nature of the stress. After a period of starvation this 50 g/day deficit must be made up, plus the protein losses required for the inflammatory response, replacement of shed blood etc. The peak demand will be from the fourth to fifth postoperative day on through to the early anabolic phase. If the patient was malnourished before operation, perhaps because of early senility, this demand will start that much earlier. In these patients parenteral feeding should be started immediately after surgery. It is a matter of simple clinical experience that patients with a serum protein level which is below 5 g% before operation are much more likely to suffer from a dehiscence of their surgical wound in the postoperative period than if the preoperative serum protein level was normal. Such patients also withstand the second anaesthetic (for the repair of the dehiscence) very badly.

ENERGY CONSIDERATIONS

It is worth calculating the energy requirements of the patient. After major surgery the energy demands are of the order of 2500–3000 calories per day plus 10% per °C for each degree of any postoperative temperature elevation. Since protein synthesis is rarely exothermic, this energy is consumed in part for the chemical reactions necessary for protein synthesis and tissue growth, blood, granulation tissue etc. Other parts of this energy are used in increased tissue activity, e.g. muscle activity such as the increased tonus of the muscles around the injured part of the body. The work of breathing may increase, particularly if there is rapid shallow breathing or partially occluded airways from sputum retention. Sweating induces energy loss from evaporation. It should not be forgotten that any amino-acid used in protein synthesis is not contributing to the fuel consumption. It is logical, therefore, not to count the energy content of amino-acid infusion when considering the energy needs of the patient if that infusion is properly balanced.

Energy sources

Intravenous fat emulsions have an energy content of 1 cal per ml. Five per cent dextrose solution has an energy content that is a quarter of this. Twenty per cent glucose solution has the same energy content as fat emulsion. In order to achieve a calorific intake of 2000 cal intravenously requires a 2 l input of 20% glucose. This volume leaves very little room for the volume of amino-acid or protein infusion. This problem is exacerbated if there is fluid restriction because of renal failure. If hypertonic glucose solutions are used, the glucose must be driven into the cells by an insulin and potassium mixture, otherwise cellular dehydration, including cerebral dehydration, will result. The overloaded circulation will then off-load this to the kidneys for elimination and this will carry much of the hypertonic glucose with it. The net result is loss of water and loss of some of the energy input.

Energy reduction

Since the increase in metabolic rate and energy consumption produced by fever is so great, all elevations of temperature should be identified and the causes treated vigorously. There should be little hesitation in starting forced surface cooling. Another way of reducing the metabolic rate is to paralyse the patient and artificially ventilate him. This not only removes the work of breathing but also abolishes all muscle tone including the excess muscle tone around the injured part. The oxygen consumption of the voluntary muscles consequently will fall. Up to 20% reduction in energy consumption can be achieved by this, more if the patient was having rigors.

Whether, when reduced to such stratagems in order to keep an elderly vascular surgery patient alive, such vigorous endeavours are worth while or whether it is merely delaying the inevitable is a matter of debate. The prognosis in this population of patients when such measures become necessary is very gloomy indeed.

REFERENCES

Abbott W. M. (1980) Renal failure complicating vascular surgery. In: *Complications in Vascular Surgery*, p. 363. Editors: Bernhard V. M. and Towne J. B. Grune & Stratton, London

Arias I. M., Popper H., Schacter D. et al. (ed) (1982) Hepatic protein synthesis and its regulation. In: *The Liver, Biology and Pathology*, p. 103. Raven Press, New York

Arunasalam K., Davenport H. T., Painter S. et al. (1983) Ventilatory responses to morphine in young and old subjects. *Anaesthesia* 38, 529

Baue A. E. (1983) Multiple systems failure. In: *Manual of Preoperative and*

Postoperative Care, p. 256. Editors: Dudrick S. J., Baue A. E., Eiseman B. et al., American College of Surgeons. Saunders, London

Bay J., Nunn J. F. and Prys-Roberts C. (1968) Factors influencing arterial Po_2 during recovery from anaesthesia. *Br. J. Anaesth.* **40**, 398

Bernatz P. E. (1906) Necrosis of colon following resection for abdominal aortic aneurysms. *Arch. Surg.* **81**, 373

Bonnet F., Harari A., Thibonnier M. et al. (1982) Suppression of ADH hypersecretion during surgery by extradural anaesthesia. *Br. J. Anaesth.* **54**, 29

Campbell E. J. M., Westlake E. H. and Cherniak R. M. (1957) Simple methods of estimating oxygen consumption and efficiency of the muscles of breathing. *J. Appl. Physiol.* **11**, 303

Chakravarty T., Tucker W., Rosen M., et al. (1979) Comparison of buprenorphine and pethidine given intravenously on demand to relieve postoperative pain. *Br. Med. J.* **2**, 895

Chambers W. A., Sinclair C. J. and Scott D. B. (1981) Extradural morphine for pain after surgery. *Br. J. Anaesth.* **53**, 921

Child C. S. and Kaufman L. (1985) Effects of intrathecal diamorphine on the adrenocortical, hyperglycaemic and cardiovascular responses to major colonic surgery. *Br. J. Anaesth.* **57**, 389

Christensen P., Brandt M. R., Rem J. et al. (1982) Influence of extradural morphine on the adrenocortical and hyperglycaemic response to surgery. *Br. J. Anaesth.* **54**, 23

Cournand A., Motley H. L., Werko L., et al. (1948) Physiological studies of the effects of intermittent positive pressure breathing on cardiac output in man. *Am. J. Physiol.* **152**, 162

De Almeida A. J. M. P. (1975) Some effects of inspiratory flow patterns on blood gas exchange in artificial ventilation in anaesthesia. PhD. thesis, University of Birmingham

Derrington M. C. (1985) The present status of blood filtration. *Anaesthesia* **40**, 334

Elliot F. M. and Reid L. (1965) Some new facts about the pulmonary artery and its branching pattern. *Clin. Radiol.* **16**, 193

Enquist A., Fog-Moller F., Christiansen C. et al. (1980) Influence of epidural analgesia on the catecholamine and cyclic AMP response to surgery. *Acta Anaesth. Scand.* **24**, 17

Epstein M. (1982) The kidney in liver disease: The hepato-renal syndrome. In: *The Liver, Biology and Pathology*, p. 752. Editors: Arias I. M., Popper H., Schachter D. et al. Raven Press, New York

Gamulin Z., Forster A., Morel D. et al. (1984) Effects of infrarenal aortic cross-clamping on renal haemodynamics in humans. *Anesthesiology* **61**, 394

George J. M., Reier G. E., Lanese R. R. et al. (1974) Morphine anesthesia blocks cortisol and growth hormone response to surgical stress in humans. *J. Clin. Endocrinol. Metab.* **38**, 736

Gjessing J. and Tomlin P. J. (1979) Patterns of postoperative pain. *Anaesthesia* **34**, 624

Gjessing J. and Tomlin P. J. (1981) Postoperative pain control with intrathecal morphine. *Anaesthesia* **36**, 268

Goldblatt H., Lynch J., Hanzell R. F. et al. (1934) Studies on experimental hypertension. 1. Production of persistent elevation of systolic pressure by means of renal ischemia. *J. Exp. Med.* **59**, 347

Gordon N. H., Scott D. B. and Rob I. W. P. (1973) Modifications of plasma corticosteroid concentrations during and after surgery by epidural blockade. *Br. J. Med.* **1**, 581

Gore E. and Hirst A. E. (1973) Arteriosclerotic aneurysms of the abdominal aorta, a review. *Prog. Cardiovasc. Dis.* **16**, 113

Hakanson E., Rutberg H., Jorfeldt L. et al. (1985) Effects of extradural morphine or bupivacaine on the metabolic response to upper abdominal surgery. *Br. J. Anaesth.* **57**, 394

Hassan H., Gjessing J. and Tomlin P. J. (1979) Hypercapnia and hyperkalaemia. *Anesthesia* **34**, 897

Hjortso N. C., Christensen N. J., Andersen J. et al. (1985) Effects of the extradural administration of local anaesthetic agents and morphine on the urinary excretion of cortisol, catecholamines and nitrogen following abdominal surgery. *Br. J. Anaesth.* **57**, 400

Husemeyer R. P., O'Connor M. C. and Davenport H. T. (1980) Failure of epidural morphine to relieve pain in labour. *Anaesthesia* **35**, 161

Kalchthaler T. (1978) The later years. In: *Family Medicine: Principles and Practice*, p. 717. Editor: Taylor R. B. Springer-Verlag, New York

Kehlet H., Brandt M. R., Hensen A. P. et al. (1979) Effect of epidural analgesia on metabolic profiles during and after surgery. *Br. J. Surg.* **66**, 543

Kelman L., Saunders S. J., Frith L. et al. (1972) Effects of amino-acids and hormones on the fractional catabolic rate of albumin by the isolated perfused rat liver. *J. Nutr.* **102**, 1045

Korinek A. M., Languille M., Bonnet T. et al. (1985) Effects of postoperative extradural morphine on ADH secretion. *Br. J. Anaesth.* **57**, 407

Landymore R. W., Murphy D. A., Kinley C. E. et al. (1979) Does pulsatile blood flow influence the incidence of postoperative hypertension? *Ann. Thorac. Surg.* **28**, 261

Lunn J. N. and Mushin W. W. (1982) *Mortality associated with Anaesthesia.* Nuffield Provisional Hospitals Trust, London

Marshall B. E. and Wyche M. Q. (1972) Hypoxemia during and after anesthesia. *Anesthesiology* **37**, 178

Morgan M. (1982) Safety of spinal opiates. *Anaesthesia* **37**, 527

Nunn J. F. (1965) Influence of age and other factors on hypoxaemia in the postoperative period. *Lancet* **ii**, 466

Nunn J. F. (ed.) (1981a) Oxygen levels during anaesthesia. In: *Applied Respiratory Physiology*, 2nd edn., p. 437. Butterworth, London

Nunn J. F. (ed.) (1981b) Work of breathing. In: *Applied Respiratory Physiology*, 2nd edn., p. 195 Butterworth, London

Phillips G. and Tomlin P. J. (1977) Arterial oxygen tensions in the elderly and in injured elderly patients. *Br. J. Anaesth.* **49**, 514

Pollock H. and Johnson G. (1973) Effect of acute occlusion of the infrarenal aorta on renal function. *Surg. Gynec. Obstet.* **137**, 805

Powis S. J. A. (1975) Renal function following aortic surgery. *J. Cardiovasc. Surg.* **16**, 565

Reul G. J., Greenberg S. D., Lefrak E. A. et al. (1973) Prevention of post-traumatic pulmonary insufficiency by fine screen filtration of blood. *Arch. Surg.* **106**, 386

Roberts A. W., Niarchos A. P., Subramanian V. A. et al. (1977) Systemic hypertension associated with coronary artery by-pass surgery: predisposing factors, haemodynamic characteristics and humeral profile. *J. Thorac. Cardiovasc. Surg.* **74**, 846

Stanley T. H., Berman L., Green O. et al. (1979) Fentanyl–oxygen anaesthesia for coronary artery surgery: plasma catecholamine and cortisol responses. *Anesthesiology* **51**, S-139

Thompson J. E., Vollman R. W. and Austen D. J. (1968) Prevention of hypotensive and renal complications of aortic surgery using balanced salt solution. Experience with 670 cases. *Ann. Surg.* **167**, 768

Tilney N. L., Bailey G. L. and Morgan A. P. (1973) Sequential system failure after rupture of abdominal aortic aneurysms; an unsolved problem in postoperative care. *Ann. Surg.* **178**, 117

Tomlin P. J. (ed.) (1976) *Fine Screen Filtration of Stored Blood.* Pall Biomedical, Portsmouth

Tomlin P. J. (1978) Intensive care: A medical audit. *Anaesthesia* **33**, 710

Tomlin P. J., Howarth F. H. and Robinson J. S. (1968) Postoperative atelectasis and laryngeal incompetence. *Lancet* **i**, 1402

Twigley A. J. and Hillman K. M. (1985) The end of the crystalloid era. *Anaesthesia* **40**, 860

Weibel E. R. (1973) Morphological basis of alveolar-capillary gas exchange. *Physiol. Rev.* **53**, 419

Weiner N. (1980) Dopamine. In: *Pharmacological Basis of Therapeutics*, 6th edn., p. 154. Editors: Goodman L. S., Gilman A. G. and Gilman A. Macmillan, New York

Welchew E. A. (1983) On demand analgesia. *Anaesthesia* **38**, 19

White W. D., Pearce D. J. and Norman J. (1979) Postoperative analgesia. A comparison of intravenous on-demand fentanyl with epidural buprenorphine. *Br. Med. J.* **2**, 166

Williams P. L. and Warwick R. (1980) Structure of the alveolus. In: *Gray's Anatomy*, 36th edn., p. 1262. Churchill Livingstone, London

Yap S. H., Strair R. K. and Shafritz B. A. (1978) Identification of albumin mRNPs in the cytosol of fasting rat liver and influence of tryptophan or a mixture of amino-acids. *Biochem. Biophys. Res. Commun.* **83**, 427

Index